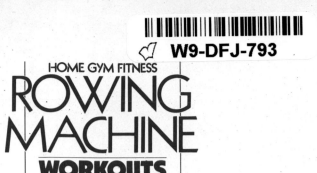

HOME GYM FITNESS

ROWING MACHINE

WORKOUTS

HOME GYM FITNESS
ROWING MACHINE
WORKOUTS

DR. CHARLES T. KUNTZLEMAN

CONTEMPORARY
BOOKS, INC.
CHICAGO

Table on page 108 reprinted with permission by *Runner's World* Magazine Company, Inc., 1400 Stierlin Road, Mountain View, California 94043.

Published by Contemporary Books, Inc.
180 North Michigan Avenue, Chicago, Illinois 60601
Manufactured in the United States of America
International Standard Book Number: 0-8092-5272-4

Published simultaneously in Canada by Beaverbooks, Ltd.
195 Allstate Parkway, Valleywood Business Park
Markham, Ontario L3R 4T8 Canada

CONTENTS

ACKNOWLEDGMENTS

The following companies provided equipment and clothing for the photographs in *Home Gym Fitness: Rowing Machine Workouts.*

ROWING EQUIPMENT

Carbos F30 and Carbos F10 Rowing Machine
Fitness Products
PO Box 254
Hillsdale, MI 49242

PROFORM 935
8170 NW Nimbus
Beaverton, OR 97005-6423

Tunturi Rowing Machine
Amerec
PO Box 3825
Bellevue, WA 98009

ROWING CLOTHES

Men's Reebok Aerobic Free Style
Reebok Shoes
2933 Oceanside Blvd.
Oceanside, CA 92054

Women's Aerobic Athletic Footwear—Princess
Aerobic Athletic Footwear
4785 Bryson St.
Anaheim, CA 92806

Women's Shirt-Short Combination
Marika Corp.
The Weekend Exercise Co., Inc.
301 Spruce St.
San Diego, CA 92103-5626

FREE WEIGHTS

Universal Weights
Universal
PO Box 1270
Cedar Rapids, IA 52406

PREFACE

IN THE SUMMER of 1984, ABC ran a special on Olympians training for rowing. Of course, athletes were shown training on indoor rowing machines. The result: a surge in rowing machine sales. In 1983, 500,000 rowing machines were sold. The Olympic year, 1984, may produce sales of almost one million. Not bad for a device that costs, on the average, about $148.

The rowing machine is all part of a dramatic revolution in the $16 billion sporting goods industry. The revolution centers on a dramatic increase in home fitness sales.

In 1984, $1 billion was spent by people like you to purchase home fitness equipment. Thirty-one million Americans claimed they had exercise equipment at home.

The reasons for home exercise equipment: costly and crowded health clubs along with Americans' passion for shaping up. Furthermore, a study Louis Harris did for Perrier, the French mineral water company, revealed that Americans want their exercise hassle-free. During the poll, this question was asked: "What would you say are the main reasons you're not getting enough exercise?" Forty-seven percent answered "not enough time," 19 percent said "family obligations," and 15 percent said "the weather." In other words, people want to look good and be healthy, but they also want their exercise to be convenient.

Some people feel that this surge in home sales is a temporary aberration. Several things argue against that point of view. First, Robert Carr, editor and co-publisher of *Sporting Goods Business*, notes, "I've seen a lot of fads in this business, but it's mind-boggling how this home fitness thing has taken off. The way these things go, it should have died out by now, but there's no sign of easing on the horizon."

Second, Thomas B. Doyle, director of information and research for the National Sporting Goods Associates, stated in 1984 that there are 150 manufacturers fighting for a piece of the hot market—an almost sure sign that the explosion of interest will continue. Diversified Products (DP) sells 15 percent of all home exercise equipment. The next-largest companies are Huffy, AMF-Whitely, Amerec, and Vitamaster. While these are the principal companies in the marketplace today, there are also many smaller suppliers and manufacturers. Furthermore, some heavy hitters have entered the field. The Campbell Soup Company has acquired the Triangle Manufacturing Company of Raleigh, North Carolina, a company that manufactures dumbbells. West Bend, a division of Dart Industries, bought out Total Gym in July 1983, and in April 1984 it purchased PreCor, a manufacturer of treadmills, rowing machines, and exercise bicycles.

Third, new products and innovations are entering the field at an unprecedented rate. Bill Stovall, president of Fitness Products of Hillsdale, Michigan, states that it is virtually impossible for competitors to keep up with what's going on in the field.

Fourth, *Chain Store Age* reports that the number of consumers who say they intend to buy exercise equipment in the next 12 months is double the number who said last year that they planned to make a purchase.

Fifth, all industry analysts say the market for home exercise equipment will increase until 1988. The average annual growth rate is 20 percent!

All the hype and attention have produced a critical mass among consumers. Trendy, upscale magazines and slick advertising pieces, such as *Sharper Image*, huckster quality home exercise equipment, making these machines almost irresistible to middle/upper- and upper-class 25- to 50-year-old Americans.

Historically, most home fitness sales have been made through chain stores—Sears, J.C. Penney, K-Mart, and Montgomery Ward. Today, many people purchase from their favorite sporting goods dealer or from a new phenomenon—a sales representative who makes house calls. Regardless of from whom the equipment is purchased, these salespeople are valuable resources. They, along with the contents of this book, will show you how to get the most out of your home fitness equipment.

Some of the most popular home equipment items are free weights, stationary bicycles and/or ergometers, and rowing machines. This book is one in a series that tells you how to get the most out of your recently purchased equipment. The series, titled *Home Gym Fitness*, includes three books that focus on the most popular pieces of equipment—stationary bicycles, rowing machines, and free weights.

In *Home Gym Fitness: Rowing Machine Workouts*, rowing machines will be highlighted. Rowing machines have been around for a long time. But high tech has transformed these machines from unstable, herky-jerky spring-operated devices into sleek, chrome-plated, hydraulic-operated products with electronic coxswains that are safe, fun, and effective.

So, read on and enjoy *Home Gym Fitness: Rowing Machine Workouts*. It will help you maximize the use of your rowing machine and reach new levels of fitness and enjoyment.

1

ROWING MACHINES

THE ROWING MACHINE has been around for a long time—since the early part of this century, perhaps even before that. It probably had its start on the East Coast, where rowing and sculling were big sports and athletes wanted something to help them stay in shape during the off-season.

Early physical culturists saw the machine's potential as a total body exercise device. In their gyms and books they recommended the rowing machine. Soon, companies such as Battle Creek Equipment were manufacturing rowers with hugh wooden "oars." Then there were modifications that slimmed down the rowing machine but provided a similar basic rowing action.

Rowing may be one of the most underrated and unknown exercise forms in the country. When people try my ProForm 935 their first questions are: "What are the benefits?" and "Does my cardiovascular system get a workout?" As a further illustration of the lack of knowledge about indoor and outdoor rowing, consider that currently only six books in print focus on rowing. Furthermore, there are none on indoor rowers.

All of this is unfortunate. Rowing can make you just as fit as running and bicycling. It will work your upper body, abdomen, and back—something bicycling and running could never do. In addition, you'll burn a lot of calories. To make things even better, there is far less chance of injury with rowing than with running. But more on that later.

While rowing and rowing machines may be the best-kept secret in the fitness industry, things are changing. In 1983, more than 500,000 rowing machines were sold. And in 1984 industry analysts were projecting sales of almost one million units. Because of the incredible surge in sales, the rowing machine has become the darling of the home sporting goods industry. Rowing machines are attractive, compact, and relatively inexpensive, ranging in price from $120 to $800.

To be candid, some people avoid rowing machines because they feel they are just for the scullers or rowers on lakes and rivers. Not so. Lots of people who can't swim have discovered rowing machines. Demand has increased, and the manufacturers have responded in kind.

VARIOUS ROWING MACHINES

There are many variations on the basic theme of rowing. Here are a few of the types of rowing equipment available:

THE T-BAR OR SINGLE ROWING ARM

This is usually the least expensive of the rowers. It has a single T-bar rowing arm, adjustable foot straps, and a seat that rides on one rail. The T-bar usually has a hydraulic cylinder to provide resistance.

Single T-bar models include:
Fitness Products Carbos F10, Fitness Products, PO Box 254, Hillsdale, MI 49242
Home Rower Model TR-100, MCA Sports, 689 Fifth Ave., New York, NY 10022
PreCor 600, 9449 151st St., Redmond, WA 98052
Tunturi Home Power Model ATHR, Amerec, PO Box 3825, Bellevue, WA 98009.

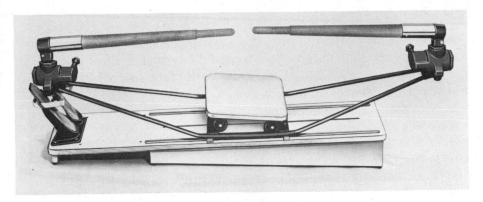

Older model wooden rowing machine.

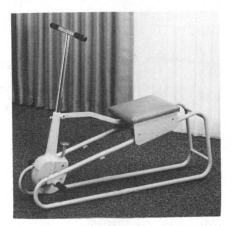

Older model T-Bar rowing machine.

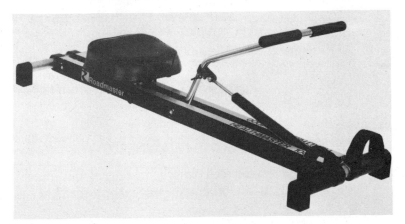

The T-bar (single arm) rowing machine is usually the least expensive.

DUAL-ACTION ROWER

These rowers are quite similar to the T-bar models. The exception is that there are dual, independent "oars." The rower has foot pedals, hydraulic- or gas-assisted resistance cylinders, and a padded seat that rides on one or possibly two rails.

Dual-action rower models include:

Amerec 610, Amerec, PO Box 3825, Bellevue, WA 98009

Avita 950, M & R Industries, 9215 151st Ave. NE, Redmond, WA 98052

Fitness Products Carbos F30, Fitness Products, PO Box 254, Hillsdale, MI 49242

PreCor 612, PreCor, 9449 151st St., Redmond, WA 98052

ProForm 935-520, PROFORM, 8170 NW Nimbus, Dept. P, Beaverton, OR 97005-6423

Roadmaster Healthmaster 1200, AMF–Wheel Goods, Olney, IL 62450

Tunturi Rowing Machine Model ATRM, Amerec, PO Box 3825, Bellevue, WA 98009

ROWING SIMULATORS

These rowers have jointed arms that rotate to simulate the dipping action of actual rowing. Resistance can be adjusted by a ratchet and disc-brake mechanism at the joint. Footrests are preset, and the seat slides on two rails. Examples of rowing simulators include:

Carnielli Super Skiff Rower, The Sharper Image, 680 Davis St., San Francisco, CA 94111

Vitamaster 901, Vitamaster Industries, 455 Smith St., Brooklyn, NY 11231

Walton 544 Rowbiciser, Walton Manufacturing, 106 Regal Rd., Dallas, TX 75247

OARLESS ROWERS WITH FLYWHEELS

Concept II introduced this type of rowing machine. It looks different from all other rowers except for AMF's Benchmark

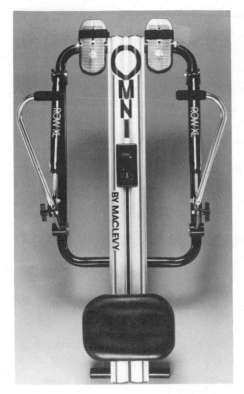

Dual-action rower, by MacLevy.

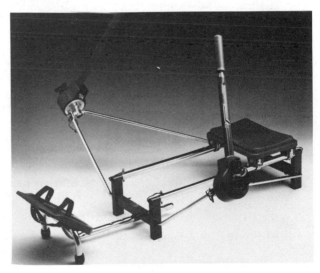

Rowing simulator,
by Vitamaster.

imitation of Concept II. Basically, this rower has a seat that slides along a single rail. The front of the rower has a wheel with plastic fins on it. Instead of oars, there's a handle connected to a drive chain that is wrapped around the front wheel. The spinning of the flywheel creates momentum for smooth action.

The stroke is started with the seat forward, knees bent, and arms extended. Then you kick back with your feet, keeping your arms straight. When your legs are fully extended you bend your arms, pulling the handle toward your abdomen, and then return to the forward position. Serious rowers say this machine comes closer to creating the feel of rowing than any other type of rowing machine.

Examples include:

AMF Benchmark, AMF-American, 200 American Ave., Jefferson, IA 50129

Concept II, RFD 2, Box 6410, Morrisville, VT 05661

OTHER MODELS

There are three basic models here. One example is rowers that tend to follow the older style of design, as shown in the beginning of the chapter. The seat slides on two metal tubes and generally moves down a slight incline. There may be one or two hydraulically operated oars. An example is *Vitamaster Model RM-6*. Vitamaster Industries, 455 Smith St., Brooklyn, NY 11231.

Another variation is the single-arm, upright rowing machine that supplies resistance on both the push and pull strokes. Pushing the adjustable handle away from you moves the seat back and down. Pulling the handle brings the seat up again. One example is *Exerow* by Battle Creek Equipment, 307 W. Jackson St., Battle Creek, MI 49016.

A third variation is the *Aerobot*, PROFORM, 8170 SW Nimbus, Dept. P, Beaverton, OR 97005-6423. This is not really a rower. The machine simulates the range of motion used in walking and cross-country skiing. The exerciser sits, so it is familiar to rowing machine enthusiasts. Yet, unlike rowers, Aerobot provides resistance in two directions.

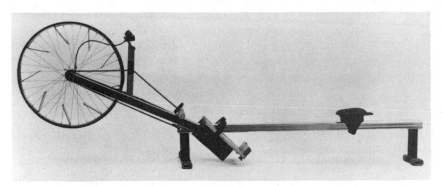

Oarless rower with flywheel, by Concept II.

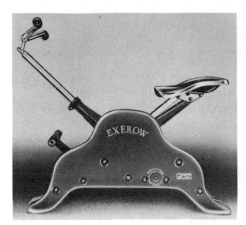

The Exerow.

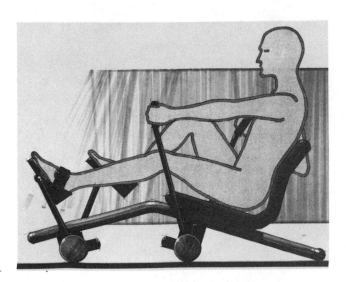

The Aerobot.

MULTI-GYMS

An innovation in rowing machines is their adaptation to mini-gyms. These rowing machines, with a few adjustments, can be used to perform a variety of exercises to condition various parts of the body.

The Octa-gym is actually a mini-gym that converts to a rower. The DP 300 and Walton Challenger are rowers that convert to a mini-gym.

Models include:

Ajay Octa-gym, AJAY, 1501 E. Wisconsin St., Delavan, WI 53115

DP 300, Diversified Products, 309 Williamson Ave., Opelika, AL 36802

Walton Deluxe Challenger Gym, Walton Manufacturing Co., 106 Regal Rd., Dallas, TX 75247

ADVANTAGES AND DISADVANTAGES OF VARIOUS ROWING MACHINES

Most of the rowing machines being purchased today are the T-bar, dual-action, and oarless rowers with flywheels. The market also seems headed in that direction for the future.

In general, the T-Bar rowers are less expensive than the dual-action models, but their quality of construction usually is not as good as that of the dual-action machines. Also, the single rowing arm means you must keep both hands on the rowing arm or do similar actions with both arms.

The dual-action model gives you greater versatility. You can adequately pump first your right arm forward, then your left arm. The dual action provides a greater opportunity to do a limited variety of exercises.

Both the single- and dual-arm rowers have one definite advantage over the other four types of rowers. They are compact and can be stored in an upright position. Consequently, your machine can be stored on end in a closet or corner of a room.

The oarless rowers with flywheels are at least eight feet long, but they do have one distinct advantage. Outdoor rowing enthusiasts feel that this type of rower so closely simulates the outdoor activity that they have organized indoor regattas in which competitors see who can row a distance in the fastest time.

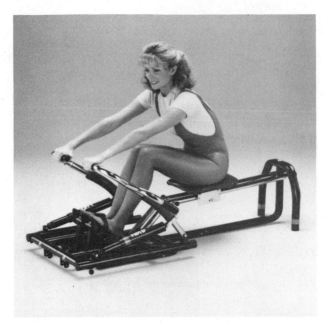

The Ajay Octa-Gym.

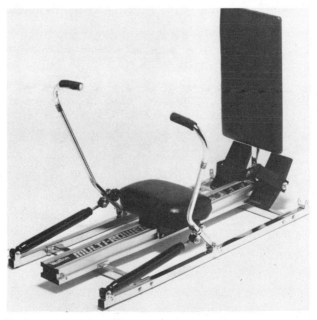

The Deluxe Challenger Gym.

The multi-gym rowing machines are a great idea. I don't think, however, that technology has caught up with all the possibilities that a machine of this type can offer. In a year or two these may be worth the extra dollars spent.

I do have a personal preference. I favor the dual-action rower, especially when just starting an exercise regimen. If, however, you are really serious about rowing and consider it your sport, go with the oarless type—Concept II. It's fantastic!

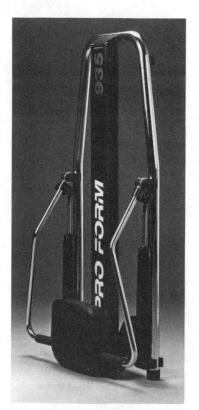

Dual-arm rowers can be stored in an upright position, thereby saving space when not in use.

2

THE BENEFITS

THE BASIC BENEFIT of rowing machines is that the exercise is aerobic. Aerobic exercises are those that get most of your body moving—exercises such as walking, running, swimming, bicycling, rowing, and aerobic dancing. Aerobic exercise stimulates your heart, lungs, and blood vessels. It helps your heart pump more blood with each beat and improves the efficiency with which your heart, blood, and blood vessels can transport oxygen around your body. It also helps you get rid of carbon dioxide more effectively.

Proper aerobic exercise produces a training effect on your heart, lungs, blood, blood vessels, and muscles. The training effect occurs 4-12 weeks into your exercise program. Some people feel the effect almost immediately, others only after weeks of regular training. No matter; we are all different and all have different responses to exercise. The rest of this chapter will describe some of the expected benefits of rowing exercise.

GOOD FOR THE HEART

Much has been said recently about how exercise benefits the heart.

For years, fitness experts have been extolling the virtues of aerobic exercise as a means of reducing one's chance of having a heart attack. The message: the more exercise you get, the less chance of a heart attack.

The heart attack death of Jim Fixx, the best-selling author on running, and the heart attack deaths of a few marathon runners have all placed a heavy cloud over these earlier claims. What is the truth?

First, let's clear up one thing. Cardiovascular fitness and cardiovascular health are not necessarily the same. Cardiovascular health refers to the health of a person's blood vessels and heart. Cardiovascular health is determined by the answers to these questions:

- Are your arteries free of fatty deposits or clogged with fat?
- Are the arteries flexible or pliable, or are they rigid and ready to break?
- Do the valves of the heart function properly, or are they scarred and leaking?
- Are the fibers of the heart muscle healthy and perfused with blood, or are they damaged, perhaps also having limited blood supply?
- Are the valves of the veins healthy, with good integrity, or are they causing varicose veins?

If your arteries, heart, and veins are healthy and/or functioning well, your cardiovascular health is good—regardless of your exercise level.

Cardiovascular fitness, on the other hand, refers to how well your heart handles exercise. It is usually determined by your response to exercise, that is, stress test, mile run, step test, or bike ride.

Usually, cardiovascular health and cardiovascular fitness go together. To maximize your cardiovascular health, cardiovascular fitness is necessary. It allows a healthy (or unhealthy) heart to reach its potential and meet extra demands placed on it.

Cardiovascular fitness may be deceiving, however. You may have significant coronary artery disease and still be able to run 26 miles or more. Aerobic exercise will improve your cardiovascular fitness and help you maximize your cardiovascular health, but the fact remains that coronary artery disease is present.

Interestingly, as you improve your cardiovascular fitness, your risk of cardiovascular disease may decrease.

With all that as background, here's what a rowing machine may do for your heart.

Your heart's job (and the blood vessels' job) is to send blood through your body quickly and efficiently. The blood carries oxygen to enable you to do a certain task. Oxygen helps your muscles to contract, your brain to think, and your organs to function. The blood also carries carbon dioxide (waste), which is eliminated so that your muscles, organs, and brain can continue to contract, function, and think, respectively. A regular exercise program on a rowing machine will improve your body's ability to transport oxygen throughout your body. How?

Proper amounts of oxygen permit your cells and tissues to work in an efficient manner. Oxygen is delivered to your tissues by means of your heart, blood, and blood vessels. When you are fit, your circulatory system becomes more efficient. That means your aerobic capacity is improved. Regular aerobic exercise on a rowing machine may:

- increase the number and size of your blood vessels for better and more efficient circulation;
- increase the elasticity of the blood vessels, thereby permitting more blood to circulate;
- increase the efficiency of exercising muscles and circulating blood so that muscles and blood are better able to pick up, carry, and use oxygen;
- increase the efficiency of the heart, enabling it to pump more blood with fewer beats;
- increase the amount of red blood cells so that more oxygen can be carried throughout your body.

These five things, plus some other complicated biochemical changes over a period of weeks and months, permit your body to improve its ability to pick up, deliver, and use oxygen. The result is more oxygen available to the tissues. The rowing becomes a lot easier.

Quite frankly, the jury may still be out on whether exercise helps prevent or slow heart disease, but one thing is clear—exercise will improve your heart fitness. It will help you get more out of life. If I were a betting man, I'd wager that regular rowing will reduce your chances of a heart attack by half. I'll take those odds!

REDUCES BODY WEIGHT AND FAT

The fat cells of your body are your fuel storage tanks. When you burn off fewer calories through activity than your body takes in, you convert these extra calories into fat. This fat is then deposited in fat cells. To illustrate this point, suppose that you eat 2,400 calories worth of food during a 24-hour period, and your level of activity is such that you burn off exactly 2,400 calories as you work, sleep, and play your way through the day. The supply and demand are equal. Your body neither calls on reserves to make up the energy deficit nor deposits extra calories in the form of fat. You maintain your weight. However, if you eat 2,400 calories and burn off only 2,300 of them, your body will convert those 100 unnecessary calories of food into fat and store it until such a time as it's needed for energy.

One pound of fat is equivalent to 3,500 unnecessary calories. Whether these calories you eat are in the form of sirloin steak, ice cream, or raw carrots makes no difference. A calorie is a calorie. With this in mind, you can see that, if you eat 100 calories a day more than you burn off in physical activity, at the end of 35 days you will have gained a pound. If you continue at the same rate, you will be 10 pounds heavier at the end of next year. By the same token, if you row for 10 minutes or so, you'll use an extra 100 calories. Assuming you are maintaining your weight, those extra 100 calories a day would mount up to about 10 pounds of fat lost in a year.

Fat is OK, provided it does not exceed 15 percent of a man's overall weight or 19 percent of a woman's. When it exceeds that range it puts you into the fat, or obesity, range of body weight.

Obesity is a subject that nobody likes to talk about. Simply defined, obesity is too much body fat. It is necessary to understand that you can be underweight, yet obese, or overweight and not obese. It sounds confusing, doesn't it? That's because we have been slaves to scales and the height/weight charts for so long that we have failed to understand the concept of lean body tissue. What we should be concerned about is fat, not weight.

Being overweight is merely weighing more than the standard-ized insurance company height/weight tables, which tell you what you should weigh. Being obese refers to the percentage of fat that is on your body. There is a big difference. For example, you can have two men who are 6'2" tall and weigh 235 pounds. One man plays halfback for the Los Angeles Rams, and the other is a less active businessperson. According to the height/weight charts, both are overweight because they shouldn't exceed 198 pounds. However, when you ask both men to take off their shirts, there is an obvious difference between the two. The professional football player has minimal body fat and a high distribution of lean body tissue. He looks very good. The other gentleman carries a large amount of fat and has very little lean body tissue. He doesn't look so good. Yet, according to the charts, both are in the same "shape."

Women usually face the problem in reverse. A woman panics at the sight of an unwanted pound. Yet, in a fight to ward off pounds, she ignores what happens to the body. Consequently, she may be at a respectable 115 pounds but move up to another dress size. She is adept at losing weight, but not fat. She has lost lean body tissue, yet gained body fat.

The key, you see, is lean body tissue, as well as the bone, organ, and muscle tissue of your body. While you can't do much about your bones and organs, you can control the amount of muscle tissue you have. A person in good physical condition will have a high percentage of lean body tissue and a low percentage of fat. A person who is unfit will have the reverse distribution.

The whole weight-loss issue now has a different twist. You need to lose fat, not weight. Unfortunately, you cannot assume that losing weight means that you are automatically losing fat. What you can assume, however, is that when you lose weight through dieting you can lose both fat and lean body tissue. Hence, you become a scaled-down version of the original model: 30 pounds lighter but still plagued with sagging muscles, protruding stom-ach, flabby thighs, and a lack of energy.

Drs. Bill Zuti and Lawrence Golding conducted a study at Kent State University to illustrate this point. The research team set out to compare the effects of several different methods of weight reduction on body weight, body composition, and selected blood measurements. The 25 women participating in the study were between the ages of 25 and 40 and were 20–40 pounds overfat. Three groups were formed: (1) Eight women were put on a diet to reduce their caloric intake by 500 calories per day, but they held their physical activity constant. (2) Nine continued to eat as usual, but they increased their physical activity to burn off 500 extra calories a day. (3) Eight reduced caloric intake by 250 calories a day and increased their physical activity to burn off 250 calories a day. Before and after the 16-week period, the subjects were tested for body weight, body density, skinfold and girth measurements, and selected blood fats.

The results indicated that there were no significant differences between the groups in the amount of weight lost. In all three groups the average individual loss was 11.4 pounds. Thus, the study indicated that all of the methods were extremely effective in controlling weight. However, the significant finding of the study was that there was a difference among the groups with regard to body composition. Those in the exercise group and in the combination exercise/diet group had undergone significant changes in body density. The dieting group lost both body fat and muscle tissue; the exercise group lost more body fat and no muscle tissue. The report concluded that, in a weight reduction program, the use of exercise is far superior to dieting alone in its effect on body composition.

When people lose weight merely by dieting they often remain flabby. If you exercise while you diet or use exercise as the means for losing weight, your muscles become much firmer. Therefore, you look and feel better after losing weight through exercise than you do after mere dieting.

The reason lies in an understanding of the fat-loss principle. Basically, there is one way to lose fat: establish a caloric deficit. That simply means that you burn off more calories than you eat. Of course, no one "eats" a calorie. We eat potatoes, meat, pies, and the rest, which contain units called calories. If the calories in these foods are not used, they are stored as fat. To lose extra poundage, you have two choices: decrease the amount of food you eat or increase the amount of calories you use.

The table on page 17 summarizes the calories used based on rowing rate and body weight.

Table 1:
Calories Used per Hour at Different Rowing Speeds

Strokes per Minute	Calories Used per Hour					
	100	120	140	160	180	200
18–22	330	375	425	475	500	550
23–27	480	550	620	590	725	795
28–32	555	635	715	800	840	920
33–35	610	720	810	905	950	1045
38–42	760	870	980	1095	1150	1265
43–47	890	1025	1155	1285	1355	1485

But rowing does more than help you lose weight and fat. It firms your muscles.

FIRMS MUSCLES

Rowing has a profound effect on many muscle groups of your body. As with any exercise, some muscles are used more than others. Here, the emphasis is placed on what exercise specialists (kinesiologists) call the *prime movers*. In a few instances the muscles called *assisters* are also mentioned.

When you start in the forward position and move your body backward by extending your legs and pulling on the levers, these muscles are exercised:

Shoulders—trapezius, deltoid

Arms—forearm flexors, biceps

Chest—pectoralis major

Back—latissimus dorsi, erecto-spinae, and semispinalis

Legs—quadriceps, gluteus maximus, tibialis anterior

When the legs are extended and you return to the starting position, these muscles are exercised (not as vigorously as those muscles involved in the backward stroke, however):

Shoulders—deltoid

Arms—triceps, forearm extensors

Chest—pectoralis major

Legs—hamstrings, gastrocnemius, and soleus

Abdominal—iliopsoas and rectus abdominis (minimally)

Rowing can be considered a whole-body exercise since most of your major muscle groups are involved.

Coupled with the number of calories used when rowing, your body takes on a well-conditioned, toned appearance. Your shoulders, chest, and arms are firmer and tauter. Your legs have better form and definition. Your waist looks smaller in comparison to your chest and shoulders.

Don't worry about muscles becoming too large. The resistance is relatively low and the repetitions high. The emphasis in rowing is on definition and shape rather than bulk and size.

MENTAL BENEFITS

Stress is prevalent. How we cope with the stresses that we are exposed to is the important consideration. Frustration, anger, and hostilities may give us high blood pressure, headaches, and other stress ailments. It is possible that a change in activity can help us master those feelings. The late Dr. Hans Selye, one of the world's foremost authorities on stress, has stated that "stress on one system helps to relax the other." Here are some examples of how exercise, specifically aerobic exercise, including rowing, can give you a mental lift.

ANGER AND ANXIETY ABATEMENT

Exercise can play an important role in helping to relieve anger and anxiety. Dr. William P. Morgan, professor of physical education at the University of Wisconsin, has noted that after a vigorous workout there is a measurable decrease in anxiety. The level of adrenaline in the blood, the blood pressure, and the heart rate are also reduced. Clinically, many people report improved feelings and less anxiety after a good bout of strenuous exercise.

While it is difficult at the present time to determine how exercise clears the mind and why it reduces anger and anxiety, it probably will be demonstrated in the future that the brain's nerve transmitters are changed in some way that causes people to feel better and more vigorous.

While I could continue to quote other people and studies on anxiety and anxiousness, I think Dr. Alan Clark of St. Joseph's Infirmary in Atlanta, Georgia, summarized it best: "It is well known that exercise is the best tranquilizer. I refuse to medicate patients with simple neurotic anxiety until they have given aerobic exercise an adequate trial." Amen!

DEPRESSION AND BLUES

Psychologists and psychiatrists are now looking at exercise as an option to help people handle the blues, or mild depression. For some reason, aerobic exercise seems to be a mood elevator. Studies done at the University of Virginia among students who claimed to suffer from depression showed that those who worked out vigorously three times a week for 10 weeks improved their scores on tests designed to measure depression. Working out lifted their feelings.

Such changes as raising a person out of depression, reducing anxiety, and transferring stress can make exercising addictive. People find that they need to exercise as much as others need their morning cup of coffee. According to Dr. William Glasser, physician and author of several books, exercise can transform negative addictions into positive ones. People often choose to give up such things as smoking, drinking, overeating, and nonproductive arguing in favor of something more enjoyable and constructive— exercise.

"I have often started out a walk in a state called 'mad' . . ." said Donald Culors Pattie. "Mad in the sense of soreheaded, or mad with tedium or confusion; I have set forth dull, null, and even thoroughly discouraged, but I never came back in such a frame of mind, and I have never met a human being that was not better for a walk." This is equally true of other forms of aerobic exercise.

CREATIVITY

Allow me to offer a personal illustration. One of the reasons I exercise is because my head calls for it. I may be happy to get the benefits derived from looking better and feeling healthier, but as far as I am concerned they are only side effects. The real reason is mental or emotional. Exercise adds life to my years. It improves my creativity. When my exercise is finished I am physically tired, but I am full of creative energy. I think I've figured out why this happens. It is time away from the phone, children, and other obligations—quiet time for myself.

A lot of times our busy schedules prevent us from taking the time for reflection necessary to the creative process. We get all wrapped up in our daily routine and do things out of habit. We know we should spend more time alone thinking, perhaps meditating, but we are filled with so much nervous energy that we can't sit still. Here's where exercise helps. The calm solitude of exercising alone gives you a chance to work things out in your mind. New ideas to help you approach old problems are more likely to pop into your head while you are rowing, running, or walking than while watching TV or worrying about that problem.

OTHER ADVANTAGES

In addition to the potential heart fitness, fat loss, muscle and mental benefits, there are other advantages of rowing.

First, rowers are convenient. They may be placed in your favorite room or office, so exercise is only a step or two away. Furthermore, they may be used regardless of the weather. Closely allied to all of this is that the rowing machine is a constant reminder to you to exercise. That is especially important in the beginning stages of your exercise program.

Second, the rowing machine has several advantages over running. Since the exerciser's weight is supported by the seat, there are fewer orthopedic problems. Therefore, the rowing machine is great for arthritics, the obese, and people with joint problems. Also, for those of us who are "normal," fewer injuries result from rowing than from running. Also, more muscles are used in rowing than in running.

Another advantage of a rowing machine is that it can be used by people with leg handicaps. Research conducted at the University of Wisconsin at LaCrosse, under the direction of Dr. Linda K. Hall, showed the benefits of rowing with the legs and seat kept immobile. Men and women were asked to row using only their upper bodies. The series of studies showed that rowing with the arms only was of sufficient intensity to produce a training effect on the body.

The benefits of rowing are many. All you need to do is set aside some time each day and get on with the joy of rowing.

3

THE BASICS

ROWING IS AN aerobic form of exercise. Unlike running, walking, and bicycling, it is also a total-body exercise working on all major muscle groups—heart, back, abdomen, arms, shoulders, and legs.

The conditioning program you select will be based on four elements: intensity (strokes per interval of time), resistance (resistance on rowing arm), duration (length of time), and frequency (number of times per week). These four elements will be discussed further in Chapter 4.

There is more to rowing than simply pulling oars. Your movements should be balanced and rhythmical. You can produce more power if your movements are efficient.

Proper form is essential to getting the most out of your newfound activity. Avoid the tendency to use your machine before you have mastered the proper rowing technique. In the beginning (for at least a week), concentrate on your form. Work slowly. This will be time well spent. Not only will you learn proper technique and become familiar with your machine, but your muscles will be given some time to adjust to the uniqueness of rowing.

For the uninitiated, the motions of rowing may seem unnatural at first. Remember these guidelines as you row:

- Do not emphasize your back when rowing.
- Pivot, using your hips.
- Allow your legs, arms, and shoulders to do the work.

THE THREE PHASES OF ROWING

Whether you are using a dual- or single-action rower, there are three basic phases of rowing.

PHASE I: THE CATCH

Come forward on your rower. Draw your knees up to your chest. Your upper body should lean slightly forward. Keep your back firm, back muscles flexed, head up, and arms straight. Grasp the oars with an overhand grip. Your chest should be up against your knees.

In this position you are ready to begin the power stroke. Keep in mind that the power part of the next phase comes from your leg muscles.

PHASE II: THE POWER STROKE

Push back against your foot pedals, exhaling as you do so. As your legs extend, continue the stroke action by leaning back slightly and drawing the rowing arms back with your arm muscles. Avoid leaning back too far—*your shoulders should not lose height.*

When your legs are fully extended, your hands should reach your chest. The power stroke should be fluid. Practice to make sure you get the action right.

PHASE III: THE RECOVERY

Since you have just completed the power stroke, it is now time to come forward. Do this by "feathering" the roller grips downward. If your rower does not have roller grips, you'll need to roll your hands anyway. Push your palms forward and thrust your wrists

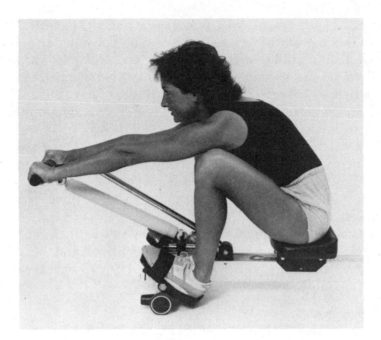

The Catch.

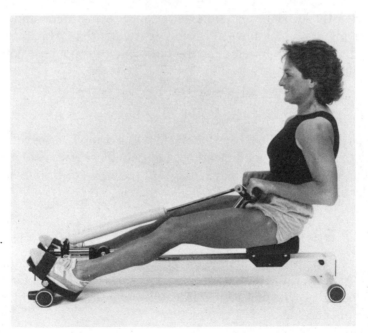

The Power Stroke.

forward. As your wrists twist, push the rowing arms ahead of your chest. This movement focuses on the muscles of your forearms.

Your arms should straighten and your body come forward. The ProForm people, manufacturers of quality rowing machines, say: "Experienced rowers use the slogan: Hands. Body. Slide. Avoid three separate movements. The transition from one movement to the next should be unnoticed.

"To master this movement, imagine someone pulling you forward by the hands. Your arms straighten first, your shoulders follow. Then your body leans forward." Your seat slides forward and your knees bend. You return to the catch position, ready to start again.

As said earlier, it takes time to master this skill. After a few minutes, review the three phases listed above and put them together. Familiarity with the machine and its movement seems to make it easier to learn the three phases.

THE THREE PRINCIPLES OF ROWING

With the three basic rowing phases established, it's time to consider three basic principles of proper adjustment and grip. While all machines have different features, the principles discussed below are common, for the most part, to the most popular machines on the market.

PRINCIPLE 1: ADJUSTING FOOT STRAPS

It is best to adjust the straps for one foot at a time. Loosen your foot strap to slide your toes beneath it. Let your heel rest comfortably against the base of your foot pedal. Pull the strap tight to secure it in place. Do not row barefooted.

PRINCIPLE 2: PROPER GRIP

You may grip the oar handle (lever) with an overhand or underhand grip. With either grip, stay loose. Grasp the roller grip handles firmly but not too tightly. If your grip is too tight, your forearms and hands will tire quickly.

If your workouts are long, vary the grip to work different muscles, balance your muscle development, and minimize arm fatigue.

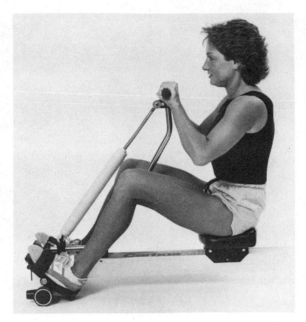

The Recovery.

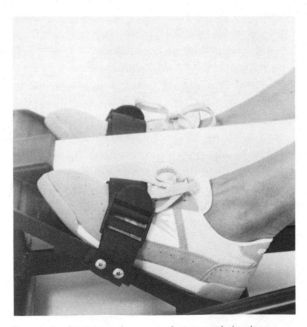

Be sure the foot straps keep your feet securely in place.

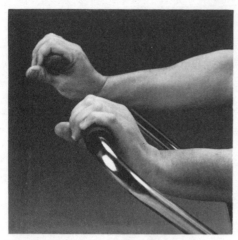
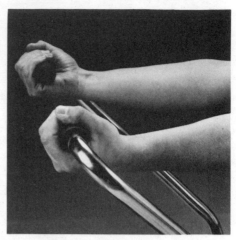

The Overhand Grip.　　　　The Underhand Grip.

PRINCIPLE 3: RESISTANCE ADJUSTMENT

There is a natural tendency to put as much resistance into the lever arm as possible. Don't. Most beginning rowers overstress their upper bodies to the extent that they can row for only a few minutes. Your goal is to row for a minimum of 20 minutes. Low resistance and high repetition is the name of the game here. Start at the lowest resistance setting and concentrate only on your form. You can increase your resistance every two weeks, as long as you stay in the proper heart rate training zone outlined in Chapter 4.

In addition to following these principles, make sure the seat is comfortable and able to support your weight. It may seem obvious, but if you must assemble your own rowing machine, make sure the seat is placed on the machine correctly. The slight rise on the seat cushion goes at the back—away from the footrests.

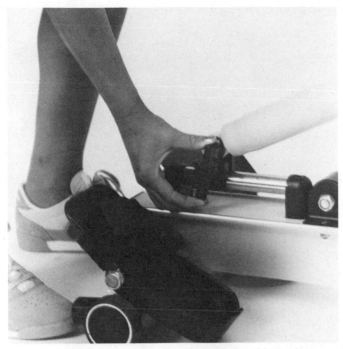

It is best to have as little resistance as possible on the lever when first beginning. As progress is made the resistance can be increased.

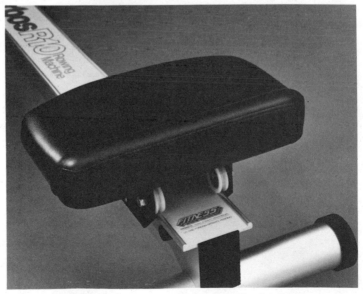

The rowing seat should be comfortable and properly placed.

4

GETTING STARTED

IN THIS CHAPTER a basic training regimen is provided for the rowing machine. The program is based on a proper warm-up, a period of aerobic exercise, and a cool-down.

This workout is designed for normal, healthy individuals. If you have a health problem (heart disease, asthma, high blood pressure, or obesity), see Chapter 6.

Before you begin, a word of caution: If you have any question about your health and have not exercised within the past year, check with your doctor. That is good common sense. Also, if you don't plan on exercising and have a question about your health, see your doctor. Your doctor can tell you whether it is safe for you to continue to be inactive.

Before we get to the actual training program, you should know something about how hard, how long, and how often you should exercise for fitness benefits.

HOW MUCH EXERCISE DO YOU NEED?

The amount of exercise you need depends on personal goals and how you perceive your exercise. Basically, physiologists talk about intensity (how hard you exercise), duration (how long), and frequency (how often). Of these three factors, most experts favor intensity as the key to proper exercise. That is, you should get your heart rate up to 130 beats per minute and keep it there for 20–30 minutes. They also recommend exercising three times a week.

While these recommendations are valid, they do not take into account that the intensity may be decreased if the duration and frequency are increased. In other words, there is an interaction among these three factors. In reality, intensity, duration, and frequency make up a fourth factor—total work. Total work is the real key to fitness and weight control.

Let me explain. Total work is a combination of how hard, how long, and how often you exercise. A minimum heart rate threshold (somewhere between 40 and 50 percent of maximum), a minimum amount of time (about 15–20 minutes), and a minimum number of days per week (2–4) are necessary for effective training. These factors can be adjusted so that, if you work harder (more intensely), you do not need to exercise as long. But the converse is also true. If you work at a lower intensity, you need to exercise longer. The charts in this book and the following sections on how hard, how long, and how often you should exercise are based on the total work concept.

HOW HARD?

The best way to determine how hard you should exercise is to measure the maximum amount of oxygen your body is capable of using. To do this, doctors have you ride a specialized bicycle or walk or run on a treadmill. While you give it an all-out effort, the doctor measures the amount of oxygen you use. Since it is a maximum effort, it is called *maximum oxygen uptake (max VO₂)*. With this information, the physician can give you a prescription for how hard to exercise.

Most of us can't afford this type of testing, or don't want to spend the necessary fees, or don't have ready access to the facilities. Fortunately, there is an alternative: checking your heart rate. When you exercise, your muscles demand more oxygen. Your heart rate and breathing speed up to get more oxygen to your exercising muscles. As you might expect, there is a parallel increase in heart rate and oxygen usage. Because of this parallel

HEART RATE

The number of times your heart pumps blood each minute is your pulse rate or heart rate. To feel your pulse, turn the palm of your hand up and place two or three fingers of your right hand on the thumb side of your left wrist. This point is called the *radial pulse*.

When taking your pulse, you should feel a push or thump against your fingers. Each push is one beat of your heart. This beat is called your *pulse*. The number of pushes each minute is your heart or pulse rate. If you have trouble locating your radial pulse, place your first two fingers on one side of your throat just below the point of the jaw and locate the carotid artery. As you do this, press lightly. Avoid pressing too hard when checking a carotid pulse.

After locating your heartbeat, look at the sweep second hand on your watch. Starting with zero, count the number of beats for a 10-second interval. Multiply that number by six. This represents your resting heart rate per minute.

Table 2:
Maximum Heart Rate

Age	Maximum Heart Rate (bpm)*
20	200
25	195
30	190
35	185
40	180
45	175
50	170
55	165
60	160
65	155
70	150

*bpm = beats per minute

increase, you can use your heart rate as a worthy replacement for the sophisticated testing. Simply reach for your wrist and count your pulse (see box). Then make sure you exercise at a level that keeps your heart beating at the proper rate. That rate will be different for different people.

Everyone has a maximum heart rate. Your maximum heart rate is the number of beats your heart makes per minute when you are exercising as hard, as fast, and as long as possible. Although it varies from person to person, your maximum heart rate is roughly 220 minus your age. If you are a 20-year-old, your maximum heart rate is about 200; if you are 40 it's about 180 (see Table 2).

Do not try to exercise at your maximum heart rate level. That is not necessary for general fitness. A safe and more appropriate level ranges between 40 and 75 percent of your maximum. That is your ideal heart rate range.

To find your ideal heart rate range, you must first find your resting heart rate. When you are rested, relaxed, and sitting or lying down, check your pulse for one minute to find your resting heart rate. Subtract the number of resting beats per minute from your maximum heart rate (Table 2). That gives you your heart rate. Then take 40–75 percent of this heart rate and add that answer to your resting heart rate. For example, the calculation for a 40-year-old who has a resting heart rate of 60 will look like this:

$$
\begin{array}{ll}
180 & \text{Maximum heart rate} \\
\underline{-60} & \text{Resting heart rate} \\
120 & \text{Heart rate}
\end{array}
$$

$$120 \times .40 = 48 + \text{Resting heart rate (60)} = 108$$
$$120 \times .75 = 90 + \text{Resting heart rate (60)} = 150$$

This person's ideal heart rate range would be 108–150 beats per minute.

To spare you all this math, simply look at the accompanying charts. All the calculations are done for you. First, locate your age chart. Then find your resting heart rate at the top of your age chart. From this you'll be able to find your ideal heart rate range for exercise.

Table 3:
Exercise Heart Rate Age 20 and Under

% of Max. Heart Rate	Resting Heart Rates					
	54 or less	55–64	65–74	75–84	85–94	95 or more
40%	110–115	116–122	122–127	128–133	134–139	140–144
45%	116–122	123–129	128–134	134–139	140–144	145–149
50%	123–129	130–136	135–141	140–145	145–149	150–154
55%	130–136	137–141	142–147	146–151	150–155	155–159
60%	137–143	142–147	148–153	152–157	156–161	160–164
65%	144–150	148–153	154–157	158–161	162–164	165–170
70%	151–156	154–160	158–162	162–165	165–168	169–174
75%	157–163	161–166	163–168	166–171	169–173	175–179

Table 4:
Exercise Heart Rate Age 20–29

% of Max. Heart Rate	Resting Heart Rates					
	54 or less	55–64	65–74	75–84	85–94	95 or more
40%	106–111	112–116	118–122	124–128	130–134	136–140
45%	112–118	117–123	123–128	129–134	135–140	141–145
50%	119–125	124–130	129–135	135–140	141–145	146–150
55%	126–132	131–137	136–142	141–146	146–150	151–155
60%	133–140	138–144	143–148	147–152	151–156	156–160
65%	141–148	145–151	149–154	153–158	157–162	161–165
70%	149–153	152–156	155–159	159–162	163–166	166–170
75%	154–160	157–162	160–165	163–167	167–170	171–175

Table 5:
Exercise Heart Rate Age 30–39

% of Max. Heart Rate	Resting Heart Rates					
	54 or less	55–64	65–74	75–84	85–94	95 or more
40%	102–106	108–112	114–118	120–124	126–130	132–136
45%	107–113	113–118	119–124	125–130	131–135	137–140
50%	114–120	119–125	125–130	131–135	136–140	141–145
55%	121–127	126–132	131–136	136–140	141–145	146–150
60%	128–134	133–138	137–142	141–146	146–150	151–154
65%	135–141	139–144	143–148	147–152	151–155	155–158
70%	142–146	145–149	149–152	153–155	156–158	158–161
75%	147–152	150–155	153–157	156–160	159–162	162–164

Table 6:
Exercise Heart Rate Age 40–49

% of Max. Heart Rate	Resting Heart Rates					
	54 or less	55–64	65–74	75–84	85–94	95 or more
40%	98–102	104–108	110–114	116–120	122–126	128–132
45%	103–108	109–114	115–120	121–125	127–130	133–136
50%	109–115	115–120	121–125	126–130	131–135	137–140
55%	116–122	121–126	126–130	131–135	136–140	141–144
60%	123–128	127–132	131–136	136–140	141–144	145–148
65%	129–134	133–138	137–142	141–145	145–148	149–152
70%	135–140	139–144	143–148	146–150	149–153	153–156
75%	141–145	145–150	149–154	151–155	154–158	159–162

Table 7:
Exercise Heart Rate Age 50–59

% of Max. Heart Rate	Resting Heart Rates					
	54 or less	55–64	65–74	75–84	85–94	95 or more
40%	94– 98	100–104	106–110	112–116	118–122	124–128
45%	99–104	105–110	111–115	117–120	123–126	129–132
50%	105–110	111–115	116–120	121–125	127–130	133–135
55%	111–116	116–120	121–125	126–130	131–134	136–138
60%	117–122	121–126	126–130	131–134	135–138	139–142
65%	123–128	127–131	131–135	135–138	139–142	143–145
70%	129–132	132–135	136–139	139–141	143–145	146–148
75%	133–137	136–140	140–143	142–145	146–148	149–152

Table 8:
Exercise Heart Rate Age 60 and Above

% of Max. Heart Rate	Resting Heart Rates					
	54 or less	55–64	65–74	75–84	85–94	95 or more
40%	89– 94	96–100	102–106	109–112	115–118	122–124
45%	95–100	101–105	107–111	113–116	119–122	125–127
50%	101–106	106–110	112–115	117–120	123–125	128–130
55%	107–111	111–116	116–120	121–124	126–129	131–134
60%	112–117	117–121	121–125	125–129	130–133	135–137
65%	118–122	122–126	126–129	130–133	134–136	138–140
70%	123–126	125–130	128–132	132–137	135–140	141–144
75%	127–130	131–133	133–136	138–140	140–144	145–148

To use these charts when rowing, check your pulse after you have rowed for at least 10 minutes. When rowing, you should push yourself, but not too hard. You should be breathing more deeply than usual and will probably perspire. The exercise should be pain-free, you should be able to talk to someone next to you (real or imagined), and the pace and rowing resistance should seem just about right.

Check your pulse for 10 seconds and multiply the number by six to determine your heart's beats per minute while exercising. Then locate your resting heart rate column (across the top of your age chart) and find your pulse in the vertical column. Look at the far left column for the percentage of maximum heart rate (fitness category). Remember that category. You'll need it in the following section. You'll notice that our 40-year-old has a range of 108–150 on the chart just as in the calculation given earlier. If your heart rate is higher after exercise than the range provided indicated on the appropriate chart, slow your rowing pace or reduce the resistance. If your heart rate is lower than the range shown, pick up your pace a bit during the next exercise session or put more resistance on the rowing lever.

HOW LONG?

When you are exercising to train your heart and lungs, most experts agree that at least 20 minutes of exercise at 60–65 percent of heart rate range is necessary. Of course, the intensity may be increased or decreased, but more on that in a minute.

If you are exercising to burn calories and fat efficiently, most experts agree that at least 300 kilocalories (or calories—experts use the number of calories burned during exercise as a measure of total work) should be burned or used when exercising to help control your body weight. Usually one-half hour of exercise is recommended with the heart rate being at about 60 percent of your heart rate range.

There are several reasons for these parameters. At rest, the majority of your energy comes from glycogen and glucose (carbo-hydrate). As you exercise, your body gradually shifts into burning fat stores. The longer you exercise, the more fat you use. Exercis-ing for 30 minutes (or burning 300 calories) seems to be the critical threshold you must reach to burn away fat and keep it off.

Of course, there are going to be people who cannot burn 300 calories in one-half hour. They find the 60-percent exercise range too difficult, so they want to back off a bit on the intensity. Instead, they find exercise at 40 percent of their heart rate for 60 minutes is more comfortable. This level of exercise for 60 minutes still burns 300 calories. This adaptation is important. .

Not everyone is able to exercise at the 60-percent level of intensity. For some people, maybe 40 or 50 percent is better or more comfortable. Therefore, they must exercise longer to adjust for the reduced intensity. The following chart shows you how long to exercise, based on pulse rates. When you are rowing, check your pulse and determine your percentage of maximum heart rate as described above. You are now able to determine the number of minutes you should exercise. Table 9 illustrates this concept.

Table 9:
Number of Minutes of Recommended Exercises
at Different Training Heart Rates

% of Maximum Heart Rate	Number of Minutes to Exercise— Fat/Weight Control	Number of Minutes to Exercise— Heart/Lung Fitness
40%	60:01–75:00	Not Intense Enough
45%	52:31–60:00	Not Intense Enough
50%	45:01–52:30	45:01–52:30
55%	37:30–45:00	37:30–45:00
60%	30:01–37:30	30:01–37:30
65%	25:01–30:00	25:01–30:00
70%	20:01–25:00	20:01–25:00
75%	15:00–20:00	15:00–20:00

For example, if you are rowing and your heart rate is at 60 percent of maximum, you should row for 30–37½ minutes; if you are rowing at 50 percent of your maximum heart rate, you'll need to row for 45–52½ minutes. Rowing at 75 percent of your maximum heart rate is necessary for only 15–20 minutes. All of these pulse rates for their specified amounts of time will cause you to burn or use 300 calories.

Just to make sure you've got it, let's review. There is a strong interplay between the intensity and duration of exercise, that is, how long and how hard you exercise. You may compromise the intensity of your exercise by exercising for longer periods of time. The opposite is also true—higher-intensity exercise for a shorter duration. So the picture looks like this: If you want to improve your heart and lung fitness, the ideal way is to row for 30–37½ minutes at 60 percent of your heart rate range. If you find, however, that the 60-percent range is too difficult or leaves you breathless, then exercise at 50 percent of your heart rate range for 45–52½ minutes. On the other hand, if you find 60 percent too easy, you may work at 70–75 percent of maximum and exercise for about 15–20 minutes. Regardless, the goal is to burn 300 calories.

One note of caution: For healthy, normal people, the training effect on the heart and lungs usually does not occur below 45 percent of maximum heart rate. I'm not sure why. Maybe, on occasion throughout the day, our heart rates go that high—going up stairs, stocking shelves, carrying boxes, or mowing grass.

HOW OFTEN?

Row a minimum of three to five times a week. Studies show that exercising this many times a week provides a reasonable and optimum frequency of exercise. Once you are fit, two to three times a week may help you maintain your fitness level, but three and preferably four or five times is best for getting into shape, losing fat, and staying lean over the long haul.

Make sure you understand this relationship of how hard, how long, and how often you need to exercise. I'm going to come back to it later.

THE BASIC TRAINING—ROWING

The basic training program is broken down into three phases: the warm-up, peak work, and the cool-down. The warm-up is 12 minutes long, the peak work is 15–75 minutes long (depending on your training heart rate level), and the cool-down is 10 minutes long.

The warm-up gets your body ready for more vigorous exercise. Since you have been sedentary, you need to loosen joints; stretch muscles, tendons, and ligaments; and prepare the cardiovascular system for more demanding exercise. Then you are ready to move into the peak period. The cool-down is intended to do just the reverse—to prepare your body for the sedentary lifestyle. Let's look at each aspect.

THE WARM-UP: 12 MINUTES

The warm-up has three phases.

Phase 1. Get on your rowing machine and row for four minutes at a minimum resistance and relatively slow stroke rhythm—about half your normal stroke rhythm is fine. This four-minute preparation time will increase your body temperature a bit. Your muscles will be "heated up" so that you will be able to stretch properly.

Phase 2. Get off your rower and do the following stretches for four minutes.

With the seven stretches, follow these guidelines: Stretch to the point where you feel a tug. Hold that position and visualize that the muscles being stretched are relaxing. When they seem to be looser, stretch further until you feel the tug. Hold that position for 10 seconds. Then return. Over the weeks, gradually increase your hold time to 30 seconds.

Biceps and Pectoral Stretch
Stretches the muscles on the front of your upper arm and the chest.
1. Stand beside a wall. Place the arm closest to the wall against the wall surface.
2. Slowly turn away from the wall, keeping the arm straight.
3. Hold.
4. Repeat with the other arm.

Kneeling Shoulder Stretch
1. Kneel on the floor, sit back on your heels, and lock your knees as you reach forward with your hands.
2. Keep your seat down and continue to focus on your knees.
3. Once you have reached as far as possible, press down against the floor with your hands.
4. You will feel your shoulders stretch. Hold and repeat.

Reach for the Sky
Stretches the upper back and the shoulders.
1. Kneel with the hands clasped behind the back and your seat resting on your heels.
2. Place your forehead on the ground at the knees.
3. Raise your hands above your back and head as high as possible.
4. Hold and repeat.

Cross-Leg Hamstring Stretch
Stretches the hamstring muscles.
1. Sit on the floor with one leg straight. Cross the other leg over the top of the straight leg. (This helps stabilize the leg and prevent you from bending during the stretch.)
2. Place both hands on the straight leg and, bending slowly from the waist, walk your fingers down the leg as far as possible.
3. Hold.
4. Repeat with the other leg.

Sitting Stretch
Beneficial to the muscles of the lower back and those behind the thighs (hamstrings).
1. Sit on the floor with your legs extended.
2. Bend slowly at the waist and bring your head as close to the knees as possible. Keep your legs extended and your head down.
3. Try to touch your toes and hold. This stretch should be done slowly.
4. Repeat.

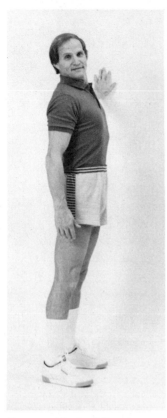

Biceps and Pectoral Stretch.

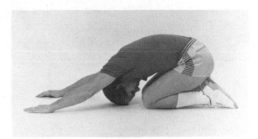

Kneeling Shoulder Stretch.

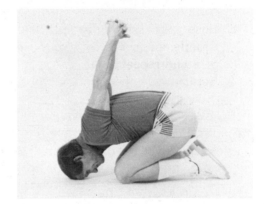

Reach for the Sky.

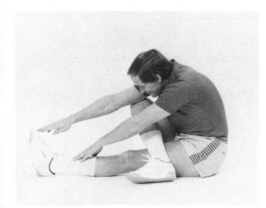

Cross-Leg Hamstring Stretch.

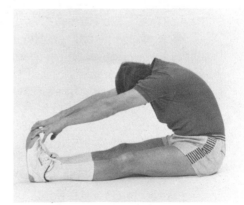

Sitting Stretch.

Sitting Ankle Rotation
Stretches the muscles of the ankles.
1. Sit on the floor, raise one foot, and support it with one hand at the calf and the other hand at the foot.
2. Slowly rotate your ankle clockwise.
3. Rotate the ankle counterclockwise through a complete range of motion.
4. Repeat several times in each direction with each foot.

Quadricep Stretch
Stretches the quadriceps muscles.
1. Lie on left side, legs extended, head resting in palm of left hand.
2. Bend your right leg so your foot comes toward your buttocks. Grasp your instep with your right hand and tug.
3. Stretch and hold.
4. Return and repeat on the other side.

Phase 3. Get back on your rower and row again for four minutes. Resistance should be minimal. The stroke rate should be three-quarters of your peak work rate.

THE PEAK AEROBIC PHASE

After the warm-up, check your pulse rate for 10 seconds and multiply that rate by six. It should be about 30 beats higher than it was when you started.

Since everyone has a different fitness level, the following gradual training approach is recommended for the peak aerobic phase of your rowing.

Week 1. Row for five to seven minutes at a heart rate that does not exceed the following:

20 years and under—115 bpm
20–29 years—111 bpm
30–39 years—105 bpm
40–49 years—100 bpm
50–59 years—100 bpm
60+ years—95 bpm

Do a minimum of three times a week. Do not push yourself; row to get a feel for rowing. You will need to experiment with rate and resistance to elicit the above heart rate. While everyone is differ-

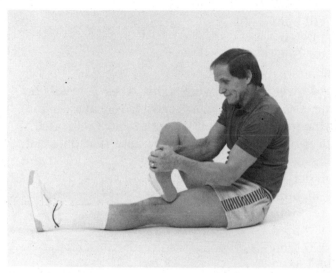

Sitting Ankle Rotations.

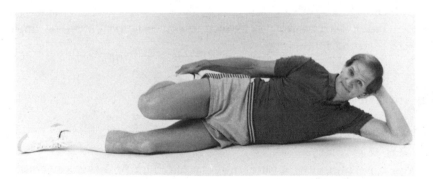

Quadricep Stretch.

ent, you might start with a rowing rate of 20 strokes per minute and a resistance of 1 or 1½.

Week 2. Row for 7-10 minutes at a heart rate that does not exceed the following:

20 years and under—120 bpm
20-29 years—115 bpm
30-39 years—110 bpm
40-19 years—105 bpm
50-59 years—105 bpm
60+ years—100 bpm

Do a minimum of three times a week. This week you will be pushing yourself harder, but again, don't strive to row at a certain rate. Just try to work so you approach the pulse rates indicated.

Week 3. Row for 10-13 minutes at a heart rate that does not exceed the following:

20 years and under—125 bpm
20-29 years—120 bpm
30-39 years—115 bpm
40-49 years—110 bpm
50-59 years—110 bpm
60+ years—105 bpm

Do a minimum of three to four times a week. Again, you are going to be pushing yourself a little harder this week, but do not exceed those pulse rates.

Week 4. Row for 13-15 minutes at a heart rate that does not exceed the following:

20 years and under—130 bpm
20-29 years—125 bpm
30-39 years—120 bpm
40-49 years—115 bpm
50-59 years—115 bpm
60+ years—110 bpm

Do a minimum of four times a week. This four-week preparation plan will get your cardiovascular system and your back, arm, shoulder, and leg muscles ready for more demanding exercise.

Week 5. Row for 15-20 minutes at a heart rate that does not exceed those listed for Week 4.

Week 6. Row for 20-25 minutes at a heart rate that does not exceed those listed for Week 4.

In the event that your body doesn't seem ready for more

demanding exercise, stay at Week 6 level for several more weeks until your body calls for more demanding exercise.

Week 7 and on. Now you are ready to get into the swing of things. Your arms, back, legs, and cardiovascular system should be ready to handle your ideal heart rate range. You are now ready to go back to the principles we talked about at the beginning of this chapter.

On the first rowing day of the seventh week, go through your normal warm-up for 12 minutes. After this, row for at least 10 minutes. While rowing, push yourself, but not too hard. You should be breathing more deeply than when at rest or during the warm-up, your heart rate should be quicker, and you should be perspiring. The exercise should be pain-free, and you should be able to talk to someone (real or imagined) next to you. You should also feel as though you could continue for at least another 20 minutes at this exercise level. Finally, the exercise should seem just right— exhilarating.

Stop after 10 minutes and *immediately* check your pulse for 10 seconds. Take that figure and multiply the number by six to determine your heart rate when exercising. Then check Tables 3– 8 on pages 33–35. Locate your resting heart rate column across the top and find your exercise pulse in the vertical column. After you have located your exercise heart rate, look at the far left column for the percentage of maximum heart rate. Below (Table 10) is an example for a 40-year-old with a resting heart rate of 70 and a just-completed exercise heart rate of 135. He or she is working at 60 percent of the maximum heart rate.

Table 10:
Sample Heart Rate Figures

% of Heart Rate	Exercise Heart Rate Resting HR = 70
40%	110–114
45%	115–120
50%	121–125
55%	126–130
60%	131–136
65%	137–142
70%	143–148
75%	149–154

Our hypothetical 40-year-old had a heart rate of 135 after exercising, which means he or she reached 60 percent of maximum. Once you have determined what percentage of maximum heart rate you reached after exercising, turn to Table 9. Find your percentage of maximum heart rate in the left-hand column and then check that row to determine how long to row for either fat control or heart/lung fitness. Whether the goal was fat control or heart/lung fitness, our 40-year-old would row for 30–37½ minutes at 60 percent of maximum. It is wise to start on the low end of the time range and, over the next three or four weeks, progress to the high end.

The number of days you should exercise also depends on your goal: cardiovascular fitness or weight and fitness control. If it's cardiovascular fitness, three times a week is the minimum. For weight control and fitness, four times a week is your minimum.

Using the 40-year-old who is exercising for weight and fat control as an example, he or she would exercise at a heart rate range of 131–136 beats per minute (60 percent of maximum) for 30–37½ minutes four times a week. The workouts should be done every other day: Monday/Wednesday/Friday/Sunday or Tuesday/Thursday/Saturday/Monday.

Stick with the appropriate intensity of exercise daily. Record the stroke rate. Keep a diary. In the appendix of this book, you will find space for recording the information. These daily records will give you a measure of improvement or lack thereof, so you can monitor progress, stroke rate, and resistance with or without a corresponding increase in exercise pulse rate.

Over the weeks, your fitness level and tolerance to exercise will improve. Every four weeks you should retest yourself. After warming up, row for 10 minutes and at a rate that seems "right" for you. Check your pulse and redefine your workout rate.

Most people will stay at the same level (percentage of maximum heart rate), except for those who were below 55 percent of maximum heart rate level. As the weeks progress, and they get into better shape, these people usually are able to tolerate higher work loads, so they increase their exercise intensity. Therefore, the more fit you become and the higher level of exercise you are able to do, the fewer minutes you will need to spend exercising, as dictated by the total work phenomenon defined earlier. Working at 55 percent of your maximum heart rate for 45 minutes, you use the same amount of energy as working at 65 percent of your maximum heart rate for 30 minutes. All the combinations of intensity and duration shown in Table 9 will result in your expending 300 calories.

Remember: Exercise levels are not provided for 40–45 percent of maximum heart rate for cardiovascular fitness since the threshold for the training of your heart and lungs appears to be at 50 percent.

COOL-DOWN: 10 MINUTES

After your peak work phase, it is time to cool down. The cool-down phase is as follows: Spend five minutes after the peak work rowing slower at a decreased resistance. Allow your body to recover. Stopping suddenly may cause some light-headedness, so row at a slower pace—maybe one-half to three-quarters of what you have been rowing. For example, if you have been rowing at 20 strokes per minute, you should slow down to 10–12 per minute.

After the five minutes of easy rowing, stop rowing and do the following stretches. With all of these stretches, follow the same guidelines as set forth for the warm-up stretches; that is, stretch to the point where you feel a tug. Visualize the muscles relaxing. Then stretch to the point of a second tug and hold. Do a minimum of 5 and a maximum of 10 of these stretches. (If you prefer, the warm-up stretches may also be used.)

Alternate Reach
Stretches the upper back and the shoulders.
1. Lie on your back and bend your knees with feet on the floor. Place one arm above your head with your palm facing up while the other arm is by your side, palm facing down.
2. Reach in opposite directions with your arms, keeping both hands flat on the ground. Hold the stretch.
3. Change arm positions.
4. Repeat.

Double Spiral

The first part of this stretch benefits the muscles of your chest (pectoralis), while the second part benefits your upper back.

1. Stand with your hands behind your head, fingers interlocked.
2. Draw your elbows back as far as possible and hold.
3. Draw the elbows forward and try to touch them together. Hold and repeat.

Pectoral Stretch

Stretches the chest muscles.

1. Sit with your legs crossed. Place your arms out to the sides at shoulder level with the palms facing forward.
2. Press your arms back as far as possible, keeping the arms straight. Your arms should stay as high as possible; work toward keeping them parallel to the floor throughout.
3. Hold.
4. Repeat.

Ball

Stretches the muscles of the lower and middle back.

1. Sit on the floor. Bend your knees and tuck them in toward your chest as close as possible.
2. Place your head close to the knees and grasp the knees with your arms.
3. Roll onto your back and keep your body in a tight ball while slowly rolling back and forth. This exercise should be done slowly.

Lateral Low-Back Stretch

Stretches the lower back.

1. Sit on the floor with your legs folded and your hands on their respective knees.
2. Remove one hand from the knee and place the forearm on the floor beside the knee as you bend from the waist toward the forearm.
3. Keep your feet firmly on the floor and bend from the waist.
4. Hold, stretch, and repeat on the other side.

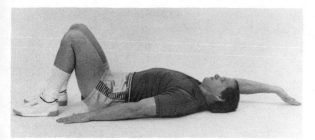

Alternate Reach.

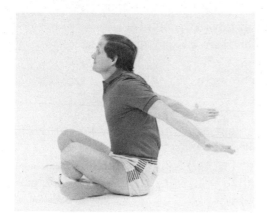

Pectoral Stretch.

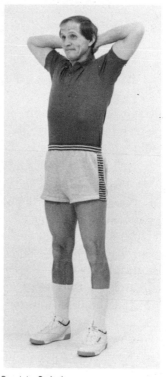

Double Spiral.

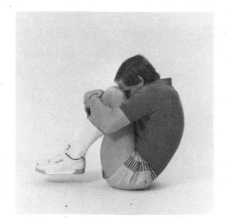

Ball.

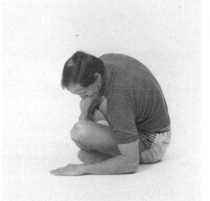

Lateral Lower Back Stretch.

Calf Stretch and Achilles Stretch
1. Stand with your right leg forward and your left leg back.
2. Keep your left leg straight and bend the right knee. Keep both feet pointed straight ahead.
3. Lean forward and slowly raise the left heel as you bend the right knee. Hold.
4. Repeat with the other leg.

Sitting Groin Stretch
Stretches the muscles of your inner thighs (groin) and lower back.
1. Sit on the floor and place your heels together. Grasp your ankles and pull the feet in toward your groin.
2. Push the knees toward the floor using your elbows.
3. Hold.
4. Straighten legs and repeat.

Shoulder Stretch
1. Hold on to a ledge or bar that is about shoulder height with your hands shoulder width apart.
2. Relax, keeping your arms straight and your chest moving downward. Your feet should remain directly under your hips.
3. Keep your knees slightly bent.
4. Hold.

Elbow Grab
1. With arms overhead, hold the elbow of one arm with the hand of the other arm.
2. Gently pull the elbow behind your head.
3. Hold.
4. Repeat on the other side.

Standing Reach for the Sky
1. Stand and interlace your fingers above your head.
2. With your palms facing upward, push your arms slightly up and back.
3. Hold, but do not hold your breath.
4. Return to the starting position.

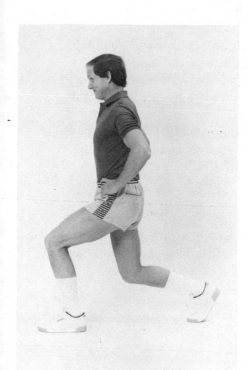

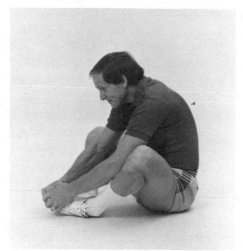

Sitting Groin Stretch.

Calf Stretch and Achilles Stretch.

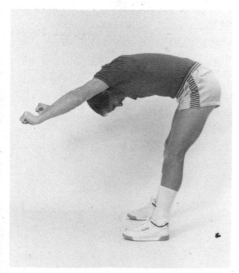

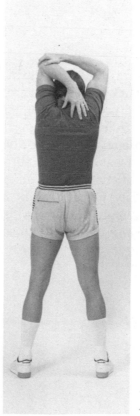

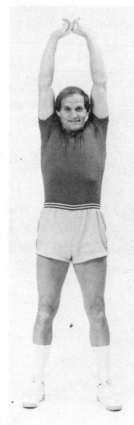

Shoulder Stretch.

Elbow Grab.

Standing Reach for the Sky.

Look Away

1. Sit on the floor with your right leg straight. Bend your left leg, cross your left foot over the right leg, and place it on the outside of your upper left thigh, just above the knee.
2. Twist your upper torso toward the left and use your right elbow to push against the left knee.
3. With your left hand resting behind you, slowly turn your head to look over your left shoulder and, at the same time, rotate your upper body toward your left hand and arm.
4. Hold and repeat on the other side.

Lying Stretch

1. Lie flat on your back. Straighten your arms and legs.
2. Point your fingers and toes as you stretch as far as you can either way.
3. Stretch and hold.
4. Relax.

TAKE IT SLOW

Don't make the mistake of slighting the warm-up and cool-down phases. Gradually working your way into and out of each exercise session will help prevent the injuries and complaints that could discourage you from continuing with your rowing program.

As a precautionary measure, always listen to your body when rowing. Table 11 summarizes the probable chief causes of and suggested treatments for complaints you may experience. Note that the majority of complaints are caused by exercising too vigorously. Remember, your goal is improved health, well-being, and fitness. Doing too much too soon will only undermine your efforts. So, as you train, carefully follow the guidelines in this chapter.

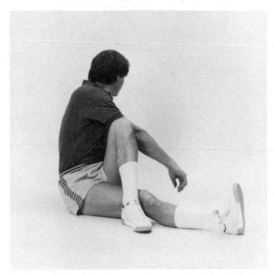

Look Away.

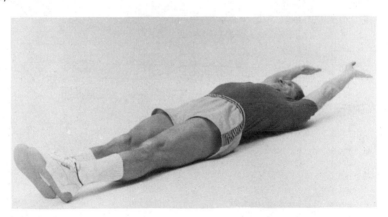

Lying Stretch.

Table 11:
Warning Signs of Rowing Overtraining, plus Cause and Treatment

Complaint	Cause	Treatment
"My heart feels funny." (This may be a hollow feeling, a fluttering, a sudden racing, or a slowing of the heart rate.)	Your rowing is too vigorous.	Slow down intensity of rowing and see your doctor.
"I have a sharp pain or pressure in my chest."	Your rowing is too vigorous.	Slow down intensity of rowing and see your doctor.
"I am dizzy or light-headed"; "My head feels funny"; "I break out into a cold sweat"; or "I almost fainted."	Your rowing is too vigorous. Not enough blood gets to your brain.	Slow down intensity of rowing and see your doctor.
"My heart seems to be beating too fast 5–10 minutes after rowing" or "I seem breathless 5–10 minutes after rowing."	Your rowing is too vigorous.	Work at a lower level of training heart rate range. In some instances you may need to work below that. If this doesn't correct the problem, see your doctor.
"I feel like vomiting" or "I vomit right after rowing."	Your rowing is too vigorous or you need a better cool-down.	Work at a lower level of training heart rate range. Take longer for a cool-down.
"I'm tired for at least a day after rowing" or "I'm tired most of the time."	Your rowing is too vigorous.	Work at a lower level of training heart rate range. Work to a higher level more gradually or you may need more sleep/rest.
"I can't sleep at night after rowing."	Your rowing is too vigorous or done too late in the evening.	Row at least 2–3 hours before retiring or ride at a lower level of training heart rate.

Complaint	Cause	Treatment
"Even though I'm rowing, my nerves seem shot", "I'm jittery"; or "I'm hyper all the time."	Too much rowing or too much competition.	Lay off the competition (i.e., working against the clock), cut back on your intensity, and/or switch to another activity for a short time.
"I've lost my zing" or "I'm no longer interested in my favorite activity."	Too much rowing or too much competition.	Lay off the competition (i.e., working against the clock), cut back on your intensity, and/or switch to another activity for a short time.
"During the first few minutes of rowing I can't get my breath."	Improper warm-up.	Spend more time on your warm-up, at least 10 minutes, until you get to your training heart rate range.

5

TRAINING FOR SPORTS

CHAPTER 4 DESCRIBED rowing programs for general physical fitness. This chapter discusses training for sport rowing. *The program outlined in this chapter is intended strictly for sport rowers and should not be tried if you are out of shape. If you have any question about your health, check with your doctor before participating in any exercise program.*

Dyed-in-the-wool rowers and scullers balk at the idea of using a rowing machine for training in their sport. As Stephen Kiesling, former Yale crew member and member of the 1980 Olympic team, said, "Rowing machines are fitness machines. They have nothing to do with rowing."

Kiesling is right. Rowing machines have a rhythm all their own. While the sliding seat and levers (oars) force you to use somewhat similar muscles, the rowing machines and sculls are different animals. Rowing machines simply do not duplicate the motion and energy requirements of sculls.

A few exceptions include the Concept II Ergometer, the AMF Benchmark, and the Carnielli Super Skiff Rower. The Concept II Ergometer has a strong allegiance from avid rowers, who feel it is the closest thing to being on the water.

A flywheel on the front of the Concept II rowing machine simulates the momentum of a boat. Plastic fan blades on the flywheel create air resistance to match the water drop on a hull. A drive chain system is attached to the flywheel sprocket and runs back to a handle. You can vary the amount of resistance by simply moving the drive chain to engage various-sized sprockets, thereby altering your leverage on the flywheel. A sturdy frame, footrests, sliding seat, and speedometer/odometer round out this rowing ergometer.

Because the Concept II uses a bicycle flywheel with fan blades, and with wind drag providing loading, the resistance goes up with speed, just as it would if you were in the water. Additionally, the turning of the fan blades pushes enough air back at you to keep you reasonably cool.

The machine is so exciting, say its proponents, that they have their own World Indoor Rowing Championships. At the Championships, you might see six or more rowing machines side by side. The rowers then row all-out for eight minutes. The winner, of course, is whoever rowed the greatest distance in the time allotted.

The AMF Benchmark follows principles similar to those of the Concept II. The Super Skiff, while it is considered better for sport training than most home rowers, operates on a home rowing machine principle.

These three machines are the best choices for use in training for sport. Although some of you may want to use the typical home rower in the following sport-training programs, I advise against it. Use your rowing machine only for fitness training. Use the Concept II and similar machines for fitness and/or sport training.

Training for sport requires that you condition your body through a program that will approximate the intensity of your sport. This is called *specificity of training.* You must pattern your training after your actual competition. If, in your rowing event, you are going to row for 20 minutes, your training should reflect and optimize that length of time and effort. Your training must match and exceed your competition conditions so your muscles, cardiovascular system, and energy systems can meet the demands of your exercise.

The key here is the proper training of your energy systems—and that is best done through interval training.

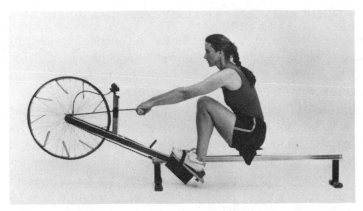

With the Concept II Ergometer you begin the stroke with your legs . . .

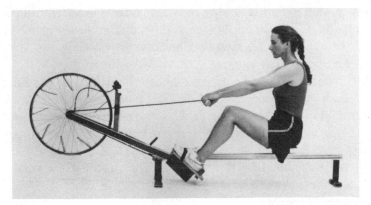

. . . your back and your legs work together through the middle of the stroke . . .

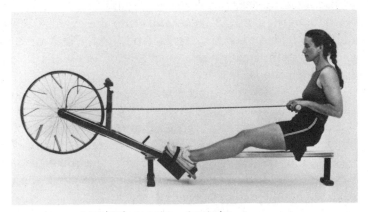

. . . and your upper body completes the stroke.

YOUR MUSCLES' ENERGY SYSTEMS

Your muscles function and do their "thing" because of an energy reserve in your muscles called *adenosine triphosphate*, ATP for short. ATP is a special chemical substance necessary for all muscle contractions. No ATP, no muscle contraction.

ATP is supplied to your muscles in three energy systems that work together to supply your muscles with appropriate energy. As you would expect, depending upon the type of the activity, one of these systems dominates. For example, when you are rowing all-out in a gut-buster fashion for 10 seconds or less, one system dominates. If you are rowing at 20 strokes a minute for 10 minutes, another system is in charge. The third system is for rowing at an intermediate rate for 2 minutes or so.

This system called into play for short bursts of incredible effort is called the *ATP system*. The long, slow, distance energy system is called the *oxygen* or O_2 *system*. The intermediate system is called the *lactic acid* or *LA system*.

When producing ATP for your body, the different systems are called upon to assist each other. That is, one system does not suddenly stop and the other take over. This interaction ensures that the systems are efficient and provide a continued supply of energy.

The ATP system totally dominates for the first 10 seconds of intense effort. At 30 seconds into exercise, the ATP system contributes 50 percent of the ATP, and the LA system contributes the other 50 percent. At 50 seconds into exercise, the LA system contributes 75 percent of the ATP, and the ATP and O_2 systems contribute the rest. At 90 seconds into the event, it's a 50-50 split between the LA and O_2 systems. And finally, at 2 minutes or more, the O_2 system is carrying 75 percent or more of the load and the LA system the rest.

Chart 1 shows the approximate contribution of each system to the replenishment of energy for the muscle, or ATP.

Physiologists say that the ATP and LA systems are anaerobic. That is, they produce ATP without oxygen being present. On the other hand, the O_2 system is aerobic. It requires the presence of oxygen to produce ATP. Without enough oxygen, the muscles are capable of only a short period of work.

Let's use a couple of illustrations. When oarsmen or women begin their race, they usually start with a tremendous burst of

Chart 1:

Percent
contribution
of system to
exercise

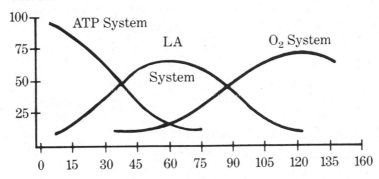

Time (in seconds) of exercise

effort and sprint through the first 30–40 seconds, averaging 40–50 strokes per minute. Here, they are using the ATP and LA systems with the ATP system dominating. Because both the ATP and LA systems are imperfect, this pace cannot be held. There is neither enough ATP stored in the muscles nor enough oxygen that can be taken in to rebuild more ATP. Fatigue starts to build. If the oarspeople keep up this pace, fatigue will be overwhelming and they will need to stop.

To prevent this, the rowers back off their pace. Stroke cadence is usually decreased to 34–38 strokes per minute. That reduced pace allows the O_2 system to dominate. The exercise, while demanding, is tolerable because enough O_2 can be taken in to replenish the ATP. The ATP and LA systems are still involved, but only minimally.

Of course, the race needs to be won. So, with a minute or so to go, the oarspeople throw caution to the wind and pick up their cadence to the 40- to 50-stroke rate. Again, the ATP and LA systems take charge in the sprint to the finish. The team or person that wins has the greatest energy reserve and the capacity to tolerate incredible amounts of fatigue. To help you understand these systems, let's consider further how they interact during exercise.

ANAEROBIC SYSTEMS—WITHOUT OXYGEN

The ATP System. An immediate demand of the muscles for ATP is supplied by this system. It taps the ATP stored in the muscles for immediate use. ATP is replenished by a breakdown of another chemical called *phosphocreatine*—PC for short. Because of this, physiologists call this the *ATP-PC system*. Although this system supplies energy quickly, the limited supply of ATP is exhausted after 8–10 seconds of all-out effort.

The LA System. This system provides ATP rapidly. It produces ATP in a process that involves the incomplete breakdown of carbohydrates. The LA system provides energy for all-out efforts that last from 30 seconds to 3 minutes. The LA system also is responsible for producing lactic acid. When the level of lactic acid gets too high, fatigue occurs and physical activity must stop.

AEROBIC SYSTEM—WITH OXYGEN

The O_2 System. This system supplies you with a great deal of ATP. If you are in good physical condition and exercise on a pay-as-you-go basis (rowing 20 strokes a minute), you can breathe deeply enough to take in enough oxygen to supply you with adequate levels of ATP.

INTERACTION AMONG THE THREE SYSTEMS

Many times in exercising, there is a strong interplay between the LA and O_2 systems. During an all-out 8,000-meter race, you will be pushing yourself beyond your oxygen limits and going to what is called your *anaerobic threshold*. The push occurs as a sprint at the beginning and end of the race.

When you are rowing easily, your demand for oxygen is supplied constantly. This is called *steady-state exercise*. But, when you quicken your pace at the end of a race and push yourself to beat an opponent, your body's demand for oxygen can no longer be met. So, your anaerobic (ATP and LA) systems kick in. Lactic acid is produced. This point is called your *anaerobic threshold*. Your anaerobic threshold is at about 90 percent of your maximum effort. Well-trained athletes condition their bodies so that the anaerobic threshold is pushed back, allowing them to push longer and harder. By raising the anaerobic threshold, they can start the sprint or kick to the finish earlier and at an even greater intensity. Between evenly matched athletes, the victory usually goes to the athlete with the higher anaerobic threshold.

If all this biochemistry tests your sanity, just remember the following:

- Your body uses three different energy systems to replenish ATP.
- There is an overlap among the three systems.
- The energy systems must be trained near their maximum (85 percent or above) to reach top sport performance levels.

INTERVAL TRAINING

Improving your sport performance in rowing often means raising your anaerobic threshold. Research has demonstrated that interval training, a series of repeated bouts of hard exercise alternated with periods of rest (usually light exercise), is the best method for both raising that threshold and simulating the demand of competition.

Interval training also has a third benefit: it allows you to do more work. Suppose you rowed as hard as possible for one minute. At the end, you would be exhausted. But now suppose you rowed intermittently. That is, you rowed just as hard for 10 seconds as you did for one minute, then rested for 30 seconds, then rowed again (hard) for 10 seconds. If you followed this pattern of rowing hard for 10 seconds and resting for 30 seconds 6 times, you would perform the same amount of work as in one minute (6 bouts × 10 seconds = 60 seconds). There would be one difference. The degree of fatigue you felt after the interval training would have been a lot less than after the continuous training. If you doubt it, try it sometime.

The reason for the difference is that hard training with intermittent rests means there is less lactic acid buildup and less fatigue. Lactic acid, as you recall, slows production of ATP. The key is rest. The rest allows you to breathe in enough oxygen to reduce the buildup of lactic acid.

The bottom line in all of this is that with interval training you will be able to train longer and harder (push back the anaerobic threshold) than with continuous training.

As you would expect, the longer the rest period, the greater the amount of ATP that is restored. According to the late Dr. Ed Fox, the following rest intervals restore these percentages of ATP.

Table 12:
Rest Periods and Percentage of ATP Restored

Rest Period	Percentage of ATP System Restored
Less than 10 seconds	Minimal
30 seconds	50%
60 seconds	75%
90 seconds	88%
120 seconds	94%
More than 120 seconds	100%

In addition, research shows that the stroke volume of the heart (the amount of blood pumped by the heart with each beat or stroke) is highest during the period of *recovery* from exercise. The higher the maximum stroke volume, the more blood and oxygen is pumped to the exercising muscles—so aerobic power (cardiovascular fitness) is increased.

In short, interval training allows you to train harder and longer than continuous training and improves your cardiovascular fitness level more. Because interval training is so intense, to do it daily or for half a year can lead to burnout. Also, interval training should not be used for improvement of physical fitness. Instead, it is to be used for conditioning and training, every other day for nine weeks or so.

Interval training is based on a series of sets of intense efforts followed by recovery periods. The training pattern looks something like this:

Set 1
Row hard for 20 seconds
Rest for 60 seconds
Row hard for 20 seconds

Rest for 60 seconds
Row hard for 20 seconds
Rest for 60 seconds
Row hard for 20 seconds
Rest for 60 seconds
Row hard for 20 seconds
Rest two minutes

Set 2

Row hard for 20 seconds
Rest for 60 seconds
Row hard for 20 seconds
Rest for 60 seconds
Row hard for 20 seconds
Rest for 60 seconds
Row hard for 20 seconds
Rest for 60 seconds
Row hard for 20 seconds
Rest two minutes

Set 3

Row hard for 20 seconds
Rest for 60 seconds
Row hard for 20 seconds
Rest for 60 seconds
Row hard for 20 seconds
Rest for 60 seconds
Row hard for 20 seconds
Rest for 60 seconds
Row hard for 20 seconds
Rest two minutes

To save space, the above would be written as:
5 × 20 seconds. (Rest 60.)
Rest two minutes.
5 × 20 seconds. (Rest 60.)
Rest two minutes.
5 × 20 seconds. (Rest 60.)
Rest two minutes.

In Table 13 is a summary of your training and recovery heart rates. These training heart rates were established by taking 85-95 percent of your assumed maximum heart rate (Table 1). The recovery rates were determined by taking 62.5 and 75 percent of your assumed maximum heart rate (Table 1). Therefore, a 20-year-old would train following these guidelines:

Rowing efforts under 1½ minutes: 166-190 bpm
Rowing efforts 1½ to 3 minutes: 166-190 bpm
Rowing efforts over 3 minutes: 166-180 bpm

The recovery heart rate would be 147-150 bpm between repetitions and 123-125 between sets.

Table 13:
Specific Training and Recovery Heart Rates
Suggested for Interval Training

| | Training Heart Rates | | Recovery Heart Rates | |
| | Training Efforts | Training Efforts | | |
AGE	Less than 3 minutes (85–95% of max)	3 minutes or more (85–90% of max)	Repetitions	Sets
15–19	171–195	171–185	151–154	126–128
20–24	166–190	166–180	147–150	123–125
25–29	161–185	161–175	143–146	120–122
30–34	156–180	156–170	139–142	117–119
35–39	151–175	151–165	136–138	113–116
40–44	146–170	146–160	132–135	110–112
45–49	141–165	141–155	128–131	107–109
50–54	136–160	136–150	124–127	104–106
55–59	131–155	131–145	120–123	100–103
60 +	Not recommended			

These heart rates mean that, if your exercise bout lasts fewer than three minutes, you should work at a heart rate that is 85-95 percent of your maximum; 95 percent is preferred. If your exercise lasts for three minutes or longer, you are to exercise at 85-90 percent of your maximum heart rate. During the rest periods between hard exercise bouts, your heart rate should drop to the repetition range. Between sets, it should drop to the set range. These decreases will ensure adequate rest so you can return to vigorous exercise.

On the following pages are two training plans. The first is for rowing events of about 2,000 meters lasting 6–10 minutes. The second training plan is for longer rowing events of 8,000 meters or more.

Table 14:
Interval Training Program for
Rowing Distances of 2000 Meters

Day(s)	Training Plans	Day(s)	Training Plans
First Week			4 x 0:40 (rest 2:00)
1	8 x 0:20 (rest 1:00)		Rest 2:00
			4 x 0:40 (rest 2:00)
2	2 x 2:00 (rest 4:00)		
	Rest 2:00	3	2 x 3:00 (rest 3:00)
	1 x 2:00 (rest 4:00)		Rest 2:00
			2 x 1:20 (rest 2:40)
3	8 x 0:20 (rest 1:00)		
	Rest 2:00		
	8 x 0:20 (rest 1:00)	**Fourth Week**	
		1	4 x 3:00 (rest 3:00)
Second Week		2	4 x 0:40 (rest 1:55)
1	3 x 2:00 (rest 4:00)		Rest 2:00
	Rest 2:00		8 x 0:20 (rest 0:55)
	2 x 2:00 (rest 4:00)		Rest 2:00
			8 x 0:20 (rest 0:55)
2	4 x 0:40 (rest 2:00)	3	4 x 2:00 (rest 2:00)
	Rest 2:00		
	8 x 0:20 (rest 1:00)	**Fifth Week**	
	Rest 2:00	1	4 x 0:40 (rest 1:50)
	8 x 0:20 (rest 1:00)		Rest 2:00
3	4 x 3:00 (rest 3:00)		8 x 0:20 (rest 0:45)
			Rest 2:00
Third Week			8 x 0:20 (rest 0:45)
1	4 x 2:00 (rest 4:00)	2	5 x 2:00 (rest 4:00)
	Rest 2:00	3	4 x 0:40 (rest 1:50)
	2 x 1:20 (rest 2:40)		Rest 2:00
2	4 x 0:40 (rest 2:00)		8 x 0:20 (rest 0:45)
	Rest 2:00		Rest 2:00
	4 x 0:40 (rest 2:00)		8 x 0:20 (rest 0:45)
	Rest 2:00		

Table 14: cont.
Interval Training Program for
Rowing Distances of 2000 Meters

Day(s)	Training Plans		
Sixth Week		**Eighth Week**	
1	2 x 3:00 (rest 3:00) Rest 2:00 2 x 1:30 (rest 3:00)	1	4 x 0:40 (rest 1:50) Rest 2:00 8 x 0:20 (rest 0:45)
2	4 x 0:40 (rest 1:50) Rest 2:00 4 x 0:40 (rest 1:50) Rest 2:00 4 x 0:40 (rest 1:50) Rest 2:00 4 x 0:40 (rest 1:50)		Rest 2:00 8 x 0:20 (rest 0:45)
		2	3 x 3:30 (rest 3:30)
		3	4 x 0:40 (rest 1:50) Rest 2:00 8 x 0:20 (rest 0:45) Rest 2:00 8 x 0:20 (rest 0:45)
3	1 x 4:30 (rest 2:15) 2 x 3:30 (rest 1:45)		
		Ninth Week	
Seventh Week		1	2 x 3:00 (rest 3:00) Rest 2:00 2 x 1:30 (rest 3:00)
1	4 x 0:40 (rest 1:50) Rest 2:00 8 x 0:20 (rest 0:45) Rest 2:00 8 x 0:20 (rest 0:45)	2	4 x 0:40 (rest 1:50) Rest 2:00 4 x 0:40 (rest 1:50) Rest 2:00
2	3 x 3:30 (rest 3:30)		4 x 0:40 (rest 1:50) Rest 2:00 4 x 0:40 (rest 1:50)
3	4 x 0:40 (rest 1:50) Rest 2:00 8 x 0:20 (rest 0:45) Rest 2:00 8 x 0:20 (rest 0:45)	3	2 x 5:00 (rest 2:30) Rest 2:00 3 x 1:30 (rest 3:00)

Table 15:
Interval Training Program for
Rowing Distances of 8000 Meters

Day(s)	Training Plans		
First Week			Rest 2:00
1	2 x 2:15 (rest 4:30)		4 x 0:40 (rest 2:00)
	Rest 2:00		Rest 2:00
	2 x 1:20 (rest 2:40)		4 x 0:40 (rest 2:00)
	Rest 2:00	3	2 x 3:00 (rest 3:00)
2	4 x 0:40 (rest 2:00)		Rest 2:00
	Rest 2:00		2 x 1:20 (rest 2:40)
	4 x 0:40 (rest 2:00)		
	Rest 2:00	**Fourth Week**	
	4 x 0:40 (rest 2:00)	1	4 x 2:00 (rest 4:00)
3	1 x 3:00 (rest 3:00)		Rest 2:00
	Rest 2:00		2 x 1:20 (rest 2:40)
	2 x 1:20 (rest 2:40)	2	4 x 0:40 (rest 1:55)
	Rest 2:00		Rest 2:00
			4 x 0:40 (rest 1:55)
Second Week			Rest 2:00
1	3 x 2:10 (rest 4:20)		4 x 0:40 (rest 1:55)
	Rest 2:00		Rest 2:00
	3 x 1:20 (rest 2:40)		4 x 0:40 (rest 1:55)
2	4 x 0:40 (rest 2:00)	3	2 x 3:00 (rest 3:00)
	Rest 2:00		Rest 2:00
	4 x 0:40 (rest 2:00)		2 x 1:30 (rest 3:00)
	Rest 2:00		
	4 x 0:40 (rest 2:00)	**Fifth Week**	
	Rest 2:00	1	2 x 3:00 (rest 3:00)
	4 x 0:40 (rest 2:00)		Rest 2:00
3	2 x 3:00 (rest 3:00)		2 x 1:30 (rest 3:00)
	Rest 2:00	2	4 x 0:40 (rest 1:50)
	2 x 1:20 (rest 2:40)		Rest 2:00
			4 x 0:40 (rest 1:50)
Third Week			Rest 2:00
1	4 x 2:00 (rest 4:00)		4 x 0:40 (rest 1:50)
	Rest 2:00		Rest 2:00
	2 x 1:20 (rest 2:40)		4 x 0:40 (rest 1:50)
2	4 x 0:40 (rest 2:00)	3	1 x 4:30 (rest 2:15)
	Rest 2:00		Rest 2:00
	4 x 0:40 (rest 2:00)		2 x 4:00 (rest 2:00)

Table 15: cont.
Interval Training Program for
Rowing Distances of 8000 Meters

Day(s)	Training Plans		
Sixth Week		**Eighth Week**	
1	2 x 3:00 (rest 3:00) Rest 2:00 2 x 1:30 (rest 3:00)	1	2 x 3:00 (rest 3:00) Rest 2:00 2 x 1:30 (rest 3:00)
2	4 x 0:40 (rest 1:50) Rest 2:00 4 x 0:40 (rest 1:50) Rest 2:00 4 x 0:40 (rest 1:50) Rest 2:00 4 x 0:40 (rest 1:50)	2	4 x 0:40 (rest 1:50) Rest 2:00 4 x 0:40 (rest 1:50) Rest 2:00 4 x 0:40 (rest 1:50) Rest 2:00 4 x 0:40 (rest 1:50)
3	1 x 4:30 (rest 2:15) 2 x 3:30 (rest 1:45)	3	2 x 3:00 (rest 3:00) Rest 2:00 3 x 1:30 (rest 3:00)
Seventh Week			
1	2 x 3:00 (rest 3:00) Rest 2:00 2 x 1:30 (rest 3:00)	**Ninth Week**	
		1	2 x 3:00 (rest 3:00) Rest 2:00 2 x 1:30 (rest 3:00)
2	4 x 0:40 (rest 1:50) Rest 2:00 4 x 0:40 (rest 1:50) Rest 2:00 4 x 0:40 (rest 1:50) Rest 2:00 4 x 0:40 (rest 1:50)	2	4 x 0:40 (rest 1:50) Rest 2:00 4 x 0:40 (rest 1:50) Rest 2:00 4 x 0:40 (rest 1:50) Rest 2:00 4 x 0:40 (rest 1:50)
3	2 x 5:00 (rest 2:30) Rest 2:00	3	2 x 5:00 (rest 2:30) Rest 2:00 3 x 1:30 (rest 3:00)

One more point: Athletes report, and researchers support the observation, that they are better able to tolerate the intensity of interval training if they have spent about six months training aerobically. That is, before the interval training begins, they spend six months running, biking, swimming, or rowing—doing what is called, obviously, *long slow distance* or *long steady distance*. This provides the athletes with what is called a *base of training*. With this base, they can do the interval work required and recover more quickly during the rest periods.

Your training schedule for your sport should look like this:

1. Season ends
2. Six months of aerobic training
3. Ten weeks of interval training on the rower prior to the start of the season
4. Season begins

6

WORKOUTS FOR SPECIAL PROBLEMS

ALL OF THE training procedures outlined so far are to be followed by normal, healthy individuals. Those people who have unique health situations must adapt their exercise regimens to their particular problems.

People with arthritis, high blood pressure, heart disease, emphysema, and/or obesity need special consideration. Here are some suggested exercise programs and recommendations for people who have uncomplicated conditions of these ailments.

As with any recommendations, check with your doctor before beginning, and take this book along. Your doctor may want to make some adjustments in the training according to your particular condition.

ARTHRITIS

A rowing machine is a good exercise product for arthritics, because weight is supported on the seat. The major joints of your body—back, hips, knees, and ankles—are not subjected to the jarring that may occur when running or walking. If arthritis pain is acute, do not row that day unless you have noticed that exercise reduces the pain. *Remember, always row when you are pain-free.* The major drawback for arthritics is that the machine sits close to the floor, and exercising arthritics may have a difficult time getting on and off the machine. Other than that, it's a good product.

ROWING GUIDELINES

Follow the rowing guidelines set forth in Chapter 4. Start with the warm-up as outlined. Then progress to the peak period. The peak period should be modified as follows: Treat the weeks as levels; that is, a level may mean one to two or more weeks. Move to the next level when your body calls for it.

The peak period should look like this:

Level 1. Row for five to seven minutes at a heart rate that does not exceed the following:

    20 years and under—115 bpm
    20–29 years—110 bpm
    30–39 years—105 bpm
    40–49 years—100 bpm
    50–59 years—100 bpm
    60+ years—95 bpm

Do a minimum of three times a week. Do not push yourself; row to get a feel for rowing. Move to the next level after *at least* one week of this training technique. Progress when your body calls for more demanding exercise. *Note:* Do not worry about your rate of rowing. Work at a level that feels comfortable to you. Finish with the cool-down exercises.

Level 2. Row for 7–10 minutes at a heart rate that does not exceed the following:

    20 years and under—120 bpm
    20–29 years—115 bpm
    30–39 years—110 bpm
    40–49 years—105 bpm
    50–59 years—105 bpm
    60+ years—100 bpm

Do a minimum of three times a week. This week you will be pushing yourself harder, but again, don't strive to row at a certain rate. Just try to work so you approach the pulse rates indicated. Move to the next level after *at least* one week of this training technique. Move when your body calls for more demanding exercise. *Note:* Do not worry about your rate of rowing. Work at a level that feels comfortable to you. Finish with the cool-down exercises.

Level 3. Row for 10–13 minutes at a heart rate that does not exceed the following:

 20 years and under—125 bpm
 20–29 years—120 bpm
 30–39 years—115 bpm
 40–49 years—110 bpm
 50–59 years—110 bpm
 60+ years—105 bpm

Do a minimum of three to four times a week. Again, you are going to be pushing yourself a little harder this week, but do not exceed those pulse rates. Move to the next level after *at least* one week of following this training technique. Move when your body calls for more demanding exercise. *Note:* Do not worry about your rate of rowing. Work at a level that feels comfortable to you. Finish with the cool-down exercises.

Level 4. Row for 13–15 minutes at a heart rate that does not exceed the following:

 20 years and under—130 bpm
 20–29 years—125 bpm
 30–39 years—120 bpm
 40–49 years—115 bpm
 50–59 years—115 bpm
 60+ years—110 bpm

Do a minimum of four times a week. This four-week preparation plan will get your cardiovascular system and your back, arm, shoulder, and leg muscles ready for more demanding exercise. Move to the next level after *at least* one week of this training technique. Move when your body calls for more demanding exercise. *Note:* Do not worry about your rate of rowing. Work at a level that feels comfortable to you. Finish with the cool-down exercises.

Level 5. Row for 15–20 minutes at a heart rate that does not exceed those listed for level 4. Move to the next level after *at least* one week of this training technique. Move when your body calls for more demanding exercise. *Note:* Do not worry about your rate of rowing. Work at a level that feels comfortable to you. Finish with the cool-down exercises.

Level 6. Row for 20–25 minutes at a heart rate that does not exceed those listed for Level 4. Move to the next level after *at least* one week of this training technique. Move when your body calls for more demanding exercise. *Note:* Do not worry about your rate of rowing. Work at a level that feels comfortable to you. Finish with the cool-down exercises.

Levels 7 and on. Now you are ready to get into the swing of things. Your arms, back, legs, and cardiovascular system should be ready to handle your ideal heart rate range. You are now ready to go back to the principles we talked about at the beginning of Chapter 4.

On the first Level 7 day of exercise, go through your normal warm-up for 12 minutes. After this, row for at least 10 minutes. While rowing, push yourself, but not too hard. You should be breathing more deeply than when at rest, your heart rate should be quicker, and you should be perspiring. The exercise should be pain-free, and you should be able to talk to someone (real or imagined) next to you. You should also feel as though you could continue for at least another 20 minutes at this exercise level. Finally, the exercise should seem just right—exhilarating.

Stop after 10 minutes and *immediately* check your pulse for 10 seconds. Take that figure and multiply the number by six to determine your heart rate when exercising. Then refer to Tables 3–8. Locate your resting heart rate column (across the top) and find your exercise pulse in the vertical column. After you have located your exercise heart rate, look at the far left column for the percentage of maximum heart rate. Table 10 provides an example for a 40-year-old with a resting heart rate of 70 and an exercise heart rate of 135. He or she is working at 60 percent of the maximum heart rate. Arthritics should stay at the 60-percent range or less.

ASTHMA

Asthmatics seem to benefit the most from training regimens that are not continuous. For them, interval training is best. Asthmatics, however, are not to work at the high intensities recorded in Chapter 6. Instead, they should work at heart rates between 40 and 75 percent of their maximum heart rate range, described in Chapter 4. Instead of rowing continuously, they should row with periods of rest.

A rowing pattern for asthmatics, after a proper warm-up, will look like this:

- *Level 1*—Row for 1 minute at 40-60 percent of your maximum heart rate. This is to be followed by a 1-minute rest. Repeat this cycle 5 times.
- *Level 2*—Row for 2 minutes at 40-60 percent of your maximum heart rate. This is to be followed by a 1-minute rest. Repeat this cycle 5 times.
- *Level 3*—Row for 2 minutes at 40-60 percent of your maximum heart rate. This is to be followed by a 1-minute rest. Repeat this cycle 7 times.
- *Level 4*—Row for 2 minutes at 40-60 percent of your maximum heart rate. This is to be followed by a 1-minute rest. Repeat this cycle 9 times.
- *Level 5*—Row for 2 minutes at 40-60 percent of your maximum heart rate. This is to be followed by a 1-minute rest. Repeat this cycle 11 times.
- *Level 6*—Row for 2 minutes at 40-60 percent of your maximum heart rate. This is to be followed by a 1-minute rest. Repeat this cycle 13 times.
- *Level 7*—Row for 2 minutes at 40-60 percent of your maximum heart rate. This is to be followed by a 1-minute rest. Repeat this cycle 15 times.

Spend a minimum of one week at each level. Do not move to the next level until you feel ready for it.

Once Level 7 is achieved, you can take one of the following approaches:

A. Increase your heart rate—that is, row for 2 minutes with 1 minute of rest 15 times. Only now provide greater resistance or row at a faster rate. Your heart rate is to be in the 60- to 75-percent range.

OR

B. Attempt to increase the number of minutes you exercise, to 2-2½ minutes. If you can row for 2½ minutes during each exercise bout, then reduce the number of repeat cycles to 12. Each week or so, gradually increase the duration of rowing by 30 seconds.

Here is an example:

3 minutes of exercise, 1 minute of rest—10 cycles
3½ minutes of exercise, 1 minute of rest—9 cycles
4 minutes of exercise, 1 minute of rest—8 cycles
4½ minutes of exercise, 1 minute of rest—7 cycles
5 minutes of exercise, 1 minute of rest—6 cycles

6 minutes of exercise, 1 minute of rest—5 cycles
7 minutes of exercise, 1 minute of rest—4 cycles
8 minutes of exercise, 1 minute of rest—4 cycles
9 minutes of exercise, 1 minute of rest—3 cycles
10 minutes of exercise, 1 minute of rest—3 cycles

Continuous exercise seems to precipitate bronchospasms among asthmatics. So you must use your own body as a guide. For each asthmatic there will be a maximum amount of continuous exercise when you determine your optimum number of minutes. Stay at that level, increase the resistance or rowing speed and work to a heart rate of 60-75 percent. Remember that your goal is 30 minutes of exercise. If you follow a 5-minute exercise period and 1-minute rest period six times, that is fine.

EMPHYSEMA

Your doctor and you must determine how much exercise you can do safely. He or she should tell you your training heart rate level. Once you know that, follow these guidelines:

- *Level 1*—Row 1 minute, rest 1 minute, row 1 minute, rest 1 minute, row 1 minute, rest 1 minute, row 1 minute. Do 3 times a week.
- *Level 2*—Row 1 minute, rest 1 minute, row 3 minutes, rest 1 minute, row 3 minutes, rest 1 minute, row 1 minute. Do 3 times a week.
- *Level 3*—Row 1 minute, rest 1 minute, row 5 minutes, rest 1 minute, row 5 minutes, rest 1 minute, row 1 minute. Do 3 times a week.
- *Level 4*—Row 1 minute, rest 1 minute, row 7 minutes, rest 1 minute, row 7 minutes, rest 1 minute, row 1 minute. Do 3 times a week.
- *Level 5*—Row 1 minute, rest 1 minute, row 8 minutes, rest 1 minute, row 8 minutes, rest 1 minute, row 1 minute. Do 3 times a week.
- *Level 6*—Row 1 minute, rest 1 minute, row 9 minutes, rest 1 minute, row 9 minutes, rest 1 minute, row 1 minute. Do 3 times a week.
- *Level 7*—Row 1 minute, rest 1 minute, row 10 minutes, rest 1

minute, row 10 minutes, rest 1 minute, row 1 minute. Do 3 times a week.

- *Level 8*—Row 1 minute, rest 1 minute, row 11 minutes, rest 1 minute, row 11 minutes, rest 1 minute, row 1 minute. Do 3 times a week.
- *Level 9*—Row 1 minute, rest 1 minute, row 12 minutes, rest 1 minute, row 12 minutes, rest 1 minute, row 1 minute. Do 3 times a week.
- *Level 10*—Row 1 minute, rest 1 minute, row 14 minutes, rest 1 minute, row 14 minutes, rest 1 minute, row 1 minute. Do 3 times a week.
- *Level 11*—Row 1 minute, rest 1 minute, row 16 minutes, rest 1 minute, row 16 minutes, rest 1 minute, row 1 minute. Do 3 times a week.
- *Level 12*—Row 1 minute, rest 1 minute, row 18 minutes, rest 1 minute, row 18 minutes, rest 1 minute, row 1 minute. Do 3 times a week.
- *Level 13*—Row 1 minute, rest 1 minute, row 20 minutes, rest 1 minute, row 20 minutes, rest 1 minute, row 1 minute. Do 3 times a week.

HEART DISEASE AND HIGH BLOOD PRESSURE

Rowing may not be an appropriate exercise for these two health problems. Research has suggested that people with heart disease may experience a higher number of irregular heartbeats doing upper-body exercise. These irregular heartbeats may be an indication that the heart is irritated by the exercise.

People who suffer from high blood pressure may also have some problems with rowing. Additional upper-body work may cause blood pressure to increase even more during exercise. Therefore, they should proceed with caution.

If you have been cleared to use rowing as your exercise, follow the guidelines established for arthritis. Stay at a training heart rate of 60 percent of maximum or less.

Both those with heart disease and those with high blood pressure should not row until they have talked this exercise over with their doctors and, most importantly, tried the rowing exercise with a blood pressure and heart check.

HEART ATTACK

Below is a rowing exercise program you can follow if you have had a heart attack and you have your doctor's approval to exercise. This program assumes a normal and uncomplicated recovery and that you don't need medication for relief of pain and prevention of heart irregularities. Your physician must establish your training heart rate. This will be done via a stress test. The test will indicate how high your heart rate may go safely.

- *Level 1*—3-5 minutes, 3 times a week.
- *Level 2*—6-8 minutes, 3 times a week.
- *Level 3*—9-11 minutes, 3 times a week.
- *Level 4*—12-14 minutes, 4 times a week.
- *Level 5*—15-17 minutes, 4 times a week.
- *Level 6*—18-20 minutes, 4 times a week.
- *Level 7*—21-23 minutes, 4 times a week.
- *Level 8*—24-26 minutes, 4 times a week.
- *Level 9*—27-29 minutes, 4 times a week.
- *Level 10*—30-32 minutes, 4 times a week.
- *Level 11*—33-35 minutes, 4 times a week.
- *Level 12*—36-38 minutes, 4 times a week.
- *Level 13*—39-41 minutes, 4 times a week.
- *Level 14*—42-44 minutes, 4 times a week.
- *Level 15*—45-47 minutes, 4 times a week.
- *Level 16*—48-50 minutes, 4 times a week.
- *Level 17*—51-53 minutes, 4 times a week.
- *Level 18*—54-56 minutes, 4 times a week.
- *Level 19*—57-59 minutes, 4 times a week.
- *Level 20*—60 minutes, 4 times a week.

If you need medication to manage your disease, adopt the following plan. The physician must establish your training heart rate. This will be done via a stress test. This program should also be supervised.

- *Level 1*—Row 1 minute, rest 1 minute, row 1 minute, rest 1 minute, row 1 minute, rest 1 minute, row 1 minute. Do 3 times a week.
- *Level 2*—Row 1 minute, rest 1 minute, row 3 minutes, rest 1

minute, row 3 minutes, rest 1 minute, row 1 minute. Do 3 times a week.

- *Level 3*—Row 1 minute, rest 1 minute, row 5 minutes, rest 1 minute, row 5 minutes, rest 1 minute, row 1 minute. Do 3 times a week.
- *Level 4*—Row 1 minute, rest 1 minute, row 7 minutes, rest 1 minute, row 7 minutes, rest 1 minute, row 1 minute. Do 3 times a week.
- *Level 5*—Row 1 minute, rest 1 minute, row 8 minutes, rest 1 minute, row 8 minutes, rest 1 minute, row 1 minute. Do 3 times a week.
- *Level 6*—Row 1 minute, rest 1 minute, row 9 minutes, rest 1 minute, row 9 minutes, rest 1 minute, row 1 minute. Do 3 times a week.
- *Level 7*—Row 1 minute, rest 1 minute, row 10 minutes, rest 1 minute, row 10 minutes, rest 1 minute, row 1 minute. Do 3 times a week.
- *Level 8*—Row 1 minute, rest 1 minute, row 11 minutes, rest 1 minute, row 11 minutes, rest 1 minute, row 1 minute. Do 3 times a week.
- *Level 9*—Row 1 minute, rest 1 minute, row 12 minutes, rest 1 minute, row 12 minutes, rest 1 minute, row 1 minute. Do 3 times a week.
- *Level 10*—Row 1 minute, rest 1 minute, row 14 minutes, rest 1 minute, row 14 minutes, rest 1 minute, row 1 minute. Do 3 times a week.
- *Level 11*—Row 1 minute, rest 1 minute, row 16 minutes, rest 1 minute, row 16 minutes, rest 1 minute, row 1 minute. Do 3 times a week.
- *Level 12*—Row 1 minute, rest 1 minute, row 18 minutes, rest 1 minute, row 18 minutes, rest 1 minute, row 1 minute. Do 3 times a week.
- *Level 13*—Row 1 minute, rest 1 minute, row 20 minutes, rest 1 minute, row 20 minutes, rest 1 minute, row 1 minute. Do 3 times a week.

OBESITY

Generally, the guidelines established in Chapter 4 can be followed by obese individuals. Usually, the obese person will feel more comfortable at a lower pulse rate. At first, the length of exercise may be difficult, but 30 minutes should be tolerable by eight weeks into the program.

If you are very obese, the arthritic program described at the beginning of this chapter is a satisfactory alternative.

These programs are only general guidelines. They are intended for people who have significant health problems, yet are able to exercise without any complications. As mentioned before, check with your doctor before you begin. Exercise is good, but your present health may require some modification of the general guidelines just given.

7

SUPPLEMENTAL FREE-WEIGHT EXERCISES

THE ROWING MACHINE is a great all-around exercise machine that conditions most of the major muscles of your body. However, some of you may want to try the free-weight exercises in this chapter to increase your muscle strength and/or endurance and to work on specific muscle groups that you feel need to be improved for better rowing.

There is also a series of supplemental exercises—squats, curls, and so forth—that some manufacturers recommend you do on your rowing machines, but these often prove to be unsatisfactory. A rowing machine is a rowing machine and is best used that way.

Some machines, such as the Ajay Octa-gym, are mini-gyms that double as rowing machines. Most of you probably do not have this type of machine, so an in-depth discussion of the supplemental exercises you can do on a mini-gym is beyond the scope of this book. The photos on page 85 will give you an idea of how the Ajay Octa-gym is used.

DP and Walton also provide rowing machines with a degree of adaptability to mini-gym use. But again, my own preference is to keep the rowing machine for rowing. The supplemental free-weight exercises in this chapter should be used to:

- round out your conditioning;
- specifically exercise different muscle groups;
- condition your body to withstand more arduous rowing.

FREE-WEIGHT EQUIPMENT

Free-weight equipment needed for the training plans that follow include fixed-weight dumbbells, ankle weights, and barbells with removables so that the bar can be used alone.

TRAINING PLANS

Choose one of the following two plans, depending on whether your goal is improved endurance and muscle definition or greater strength and muscle bulk.

PLAN 1: EXERCISING FOR MUSCLE ENDURANCE AND DEFINITION

Schedule

Three exercise sessions a week, with at least one day of rest between each session. All exercises selected (minimum of four) are to be done at each session.

Overload

Training weights are 20–40 percent of your maximum for each exercise. Therefore, if you tested out at 100 pounds for a particular exercise, you will be training with 20–40 pounds. Start out on the low side if you are unfit, on the high side if you are in good physical condition. Do the exercise 15 times, rest, and repeat 2 more times—that is, 3 sets of 15 repetitions.

Program

1. Lifting the training weight, you should be able to perform a maximum of 15 repetitions. You're not racing against time, but the repetitions must be done in a consecutive fashion. If you are able to do more than 15 repetitions, the weight is not heavy enough. If you cannot do 15 repetitions, the weight is

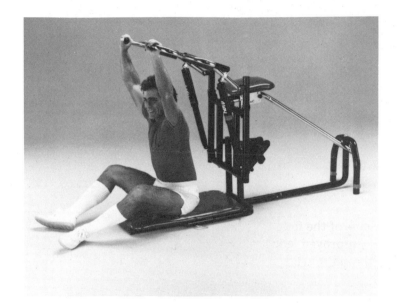

Upper Body Exercise.

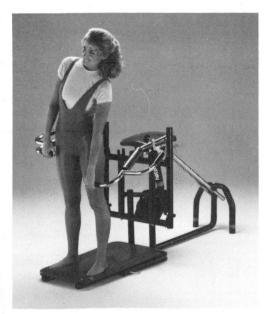

Middle Body Exercise.

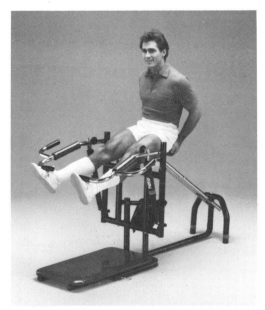

Lower Body Exercise.

too heavy. Adjust the weight upward or downward accordingly.
2. Rest one minute after the 15 repetitions. A good way to relax is simply to shake your arms and legs.
3. Repeat the 15 repetitions. No more. Because of fatigue from the previous 15 repetitions, you'll probably be able to do somewhere between 10 and 12 repetitions.
4. Rest one minute.
5. Repeat the exercise. Again, because of fatigue from the previous two sets, now you will probably be able to do somewhere between 7 and 10 repetitions.
6. After a rest of 1½-2 minutes, proceed to the next exercise in your program, following the same procedure for each exercise.

Adaptation and Progression
In one to three weeks your body will adapt to the overload of the weight and repetitions. When you can do 15 repetitions of each of the three sets for *any* given exercise, add 2½-5 pounds to the barbell or dumbbell and repeat the cycle of attempting three sets of 15 repetitions for each exercise. After several weeks, when you are able to do three sets of 15, increase the weight by 2½-5 pounds. After several months of training, the increments of increase may be only 1-2 pounds.

PLAN 2: EXERCISING FOR MUSCLE STRENGTH AND BULK

Schedule
Exercise three times a week, with at least one day of rest between each session. All exercises selected (minimum of four) are to be done at each session.

Overload
Training weights are 50-80 percent of your maximum for the entire exercise. Therefore, if you tested out at 100 pounds for a particular exercise, you will be training with 50-80 pounds. Start out with the lower weights if you are unfit, the higher if you are in good physical condition. Do the exercise eight times, rest, and repeat two more times—that is, three sets of eight repetitions.

Program

1. Perform eight repetitions of each exercise at a rate you feel is comfortable. Speed is not important. Your goal is eight repetitions, maximum. If you can do more, the weight is not heavy enough. If you cannot do eight, you'll have to reduce the weight.
2. Rest one minute.
3. Attempt eight more repetitions of the exercise. Because of fatigue from the previous eight repetitions, you'll probably be able to do only five or six repetitions.
4. Rest one minute.
5. Repeat the exercise. Again, because of fatigue from the previous two sets of repetitions, you'll probably be able to do only three to five repetitions.
6. After a rest of 1½-2 minutes, proceed to the next exercise in your program, following the same procedure for each exercise.

Adaptation and Progression

In one to three weeks your body will adapt to the overload of weight and repetitions. When you can do eight repetitions in each of the three sets for *any* given exercise, add 2½-5 pounds to the barbell or dumbbell. Repeat the cycle of attempting three sets of repetitions for each exercise. After several weeks, when you are able to do three sets of eight, increase the weight by 2½-5 pounds. After several months of training, the increments of increase may be only 1-2 pounds.

FREE-WEIGHT EXERCISES

Before you get into the exercises, be sure you understand the correct lifting procedure (see photo on page 89).

Correct Lifting Procedure: It is important that you lift a weighted bar from the floor correctly. Stand close to the bar so that when you reach down to grip the bar your shins almost touch the bar. Your feet should be hip width apart. Your hands should be shoulder width apart with palms facing backward (overhand grip). Grip the bar firmly and lower your hips and raise your head slightly, as illustrated. *Your hips should be lower than your shoulders.* As you lift, the power must come from your legs as you straighten them. Do *not* lift with your back.

Arm Press

Develops and firms muscles of the shoulders, upper back, upper chest, and back of the upper arms. Helps prevent round shoulders.

1. Stand with feet shoulder width apart. Hold barbell in front of the chest with an overhand grip, hands slightly more than shoulder width apart.
2. Extend barbell overhead until arms are straight.
3. Return barbell to the starting position. That is one repetition.
4. Repeat.

Dumbbell Row

Develops and firms muscles in the front of the arms, the forearms, the shoulders, and the upper back.

1. Stand in a short, forward-lunge position. Rest your hand on the forward thigh for support. Hold the dumbbell in the opposite hand, hanging it straight down from the shoulder.
2. Bend the elbow to bring the weight up toward the armpit, then straighten the arm downward slowly to return to the starting position. That is one repetition.
3. Repeat.
4. Repeat on the other side.

Bench Press

Develops and firms muscles of the chest, back of the upper arms, and shoulders.

1. Lie on a flat exercise bench, knees bent and feet on the floor. The barbell is supported on a weight rack or held by a partner. Grasp the barbell with an overhand grip, arms fully extended, hands shoulder width apart.
2. Lower the barbell to touch your chest.
3. Press the barbell back to the starting position. That is one repetition.
4. Repeat.

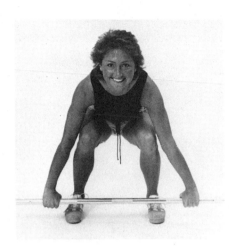

The Basic Lifting Position.

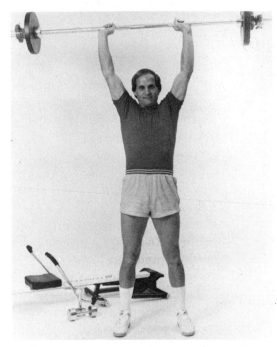

Arm Press.

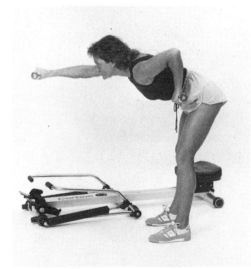

Dumbbell Row.

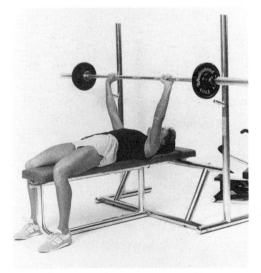

Bench.Press.

Forward Raise

Develops and firms muscles of the upper chest and shoulders.

1. Stand with your feet waist width apart or together. Hold dumbbells down at the sides of your body (or resting on your thigh) in an overhand grip.
2. Raise the dumbbells forward to shoulder height, keeping the arms straight.
3. Lower the dumbbells to the original position. That is one repetition.
4. Repeat.

Variation: Do one arm at a time.

Barbell Curl

Develops and firms the muscles of the upper arms and the forearms.

1. Stand with feet apart, arms at sides. Hold the barbell against the thighs in an underhand grip.
2. Flex forearms, raising the barbell to the shoulders.
3. Return to the starting position. That is one repetition.
4. Repeat.

Wrist Curl

Develops and firms the muscles of the forearms.

1. Sit on a bench, forearms resting on thighs and wrists extending beyond the knees. Hold the barbell in an underhand grip.
2. Extend the hands at the wrists, lowering the bar as far as possible toward the floor.
3. Flex the wrists, bring the bar upward as far as possible, and return to the starting position. That is one repetition.
4. Repeat.

Wrist Extension

Develops and firms the muscles of the forearms.

1. Sit on a bench, forearms resting on your thighs, wrists extended beyond the knees. Hold the barbell in an overhand grip.
2. Lift the bar by extending the wrists upward through their maximum range of motion. Do not lift your forearms.
3. Return to the starting position. That is one repetition.
4. Repeat.

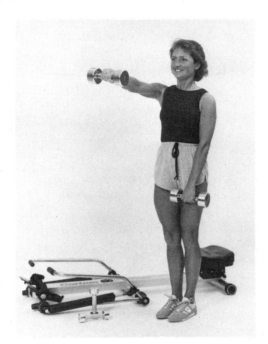

Forward Raise.

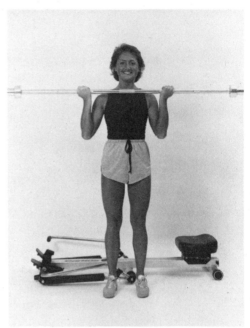

Barbell Curl.

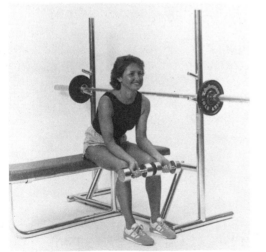

Wrist Curl.

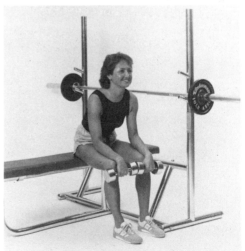

Wrist Extension.

Sit-Up
Firms muscles of the abdomen.
1. Lie flat on your back, knees bent, hands and arms across your chest. You may also do the exercise while sitting on the rower.
2. Tighten abdominal muscles and push small of the back to the floor.
3. Sit up slowly until your shoulder blades clear the floor. Stop there, hold momentarily, then return yourself to the floor. That is one repetition.
4. Repeat.

Dumbbell Curl-Down
Firms abdominal, waist, and neck muscles.
1. Sit with the feet on the floor, knees bent. Hold the dumbbells in front of the neck, elbows bent at about 90 degrees.
2. Lower your upper body backward toward the floor. Hold at this point (do not lower the shoulders and head to the floor).
3. Curl upward again until sitting upright. That is one repetition.
4. Repeat.

Note: Those with back problems should go all the way to the floor. They should avoid sitting back up.

One-Half Squat
Develops and firms the muscles in the front of the thighs and lower legs.
1. Stand with the feet spread comfortably.
2. Hold the barbell in an overhand grip behind the neck, resting on the shoulders.
3. Bend the knees to perform a half-squat (thighs no more than parallel to the floor). Return to the starting position. That is one repetition.
4. Repeat.

Knee Curl
Develops and firms the muscles on the back of the legs.
1. Wear ankle/lace weights or a weighted boot. Stand erect.
2. Curl one leg upward until your heel touches (or almost touches) the buttocks.
3. Assume the original position. That is one repetition.
4. Repeat the exercise with the other leg.

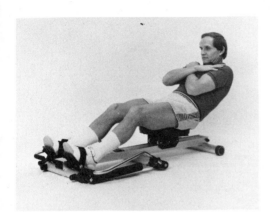

Sit-Up.

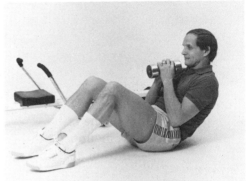

Dumbbell Curl-Down.

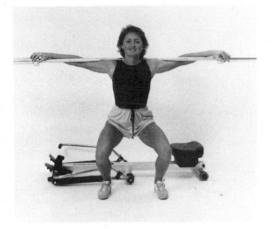

Half Squat.

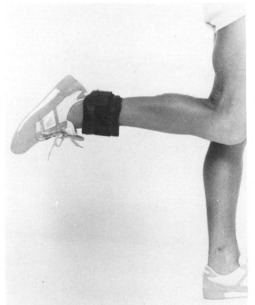

Knee Curl.

Sitting Toe Curl

Develops and firms the muscles on the front of the leg.

1. Wear a weighted boot or lace an ankle weight across your instep.
2. Sit on a table, legs hanging over the edge of the table.
3. Curl your toes upward as far as possible. Return. That is one repetition.
4. Repeat with the other foot.

Calf Raise

Develops and firms the muscles in the front and the back of the lower legs.

1. Stand with the balls of the feet on a one- to two-inch block of wood or weight plate, with the heels on the floor.
2. Hold the barbell in an overhand grip behind the neck, resting on the shoulders.
3. Raise up on the toes as far as possible. Return to the original position. That is one repetition.
4. Repeat.

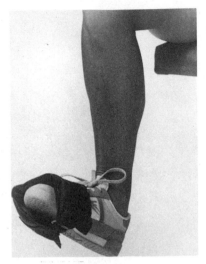

Sitting Toe Curl.

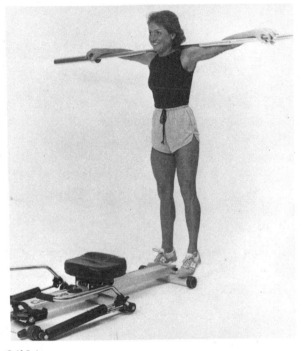

Calf Raise.

8

PREVENTING ACHES, PAINS, AND OUCHES

DESPITE THE POTENTIAL intensiveness of rowing as exercise, aches and pains are rare. Most are brought on by doing too much too soon, overtraining, and improper technique. In fact, rowing is an extremely safe exercise. Many aerobic exercisers turn to this activity after developing injuries due to running, bicycling, speed walking, or playing sport.

The three major aches associated with rowing are blisters ("the raws," in 19th-century rowing parlance), back injury, and tendinitis. While these are indigenous to rowing or sculling on the water, indoor exercisers do experience these ailments on occasion.

BLISTERS

Blisters usually occur on the hands of people who grip the "oars" too tightly, have soft palms, and/or use a rowing machine that has rigid rather than padded grips.

Blisters are collections of fluid in the outer part of the skin. They occur because of repeated rubbing against the skin in a small area. The rubbing causes the top surface of the skin to move back and forth while the bottom skin layers remain still. After a period of time, the friction separates the top and bottom layers of skin. The space fills with fluid. The top layer forms the covering of the blister. The bottom layer becomes red and raw.

To prevent blisters, you can try wearing cycling gloves, using a simple bandage when a "hot spot" appears on your hands, and avoiding a tight grip when rowing. Also, a gradual approach to training, as outlined in Chapter 4, gives time for your hands to toughen up and harden.

Medical studies suggest that blisters heal faster when fluid is drained. To do that, clean the blister area with alcohol. Next, sterilize a needle over a flame. When the needle is cool, use it to puncture the edge of the blister.

Drain the fluid by pressing the top of the blister. *Do not remove the top of the skin* over the blister. The skin helps prevent infection. Now tape a small donut-shaped pad over the blister. Wash the blister daily with Phisohex. Wear a protective covering for 7–14 days or until new skin appears.

BACK INJURY

The typical back injury in rowing is a low-back sprain or strain. A strain is an injury to the muscle belly or to the area near its attachment to the bone (tendon). A sprain is an injury to the ligament.

Since the treatments for a strain and a sprain are different, it is important to differentiate between the symptoms of the two. A strain usually is felt as a violent contraction of muscle. If you attempt to contract the muscle with an isometric motion, you will feel a pain. With a sprain, however, movement forward or to the side causes pain. On occasion, an injury can be both a sprain and a strain. One more interesting observation: sprains occur more frequently when training with weights for rowing than with actual rowing.

If you develop a sprain or strain, the RICE technique is suggested. *RICE* stands for Rest, Ice, Compression, Elevation. Rest is needed because continued exercise could aggravate the injury. Ice slows the bleeding from injured blood vessels since it causes the vessels to contract. The more blood that collects in a wound, the longer it takes to heal. Compression reduces the amount of swelling and bleeding. Elevation of the injured area, in this case the low back, above the level of the heart (lie on your belly) helps to drain the swelling.

Follow RICE for 24 hours. If pain continues past 48 hours, heat should be applied.

The Schering Corporation has listed 18 solid principles to help prevent back injuries from occurring or recurring:

1. Never bend from the waist only; bend the hips and the knees.
2. Never lift a heavy object higher than your waist.
3. Always turn and face the object you wish to lift.
4. Avoid carrying unbalanced loads; hold heavy objects close to your body.
5. Never carry anything heavier than you can manage with ease.
6. Never lift or move heavy furniture. Wait for someone to do it who knows the principles of leverage.
7. Avoid sudden movements, sudden overloading of muscles. Learn to move deliberately, swinging the legs from the hips.
8. Learn to keep the head in line with the spine when standing, sitting, or lying in bed.
9. Put soft chairs and deep couches on your "don't sit" list. During prolonged sitting, cross your legs to rest your back.
10. Your doctor is the only one who can determine when low-back pain is due to faulty posture. He or she is the best judge of when you may do general exercises for physical fitness. When you do, omit any exercise that arches or overstrains the lower back: backward bends, forward bends, touching the toes with the knees straight.
11. Wear shoes with moderate heels, all about the same height. Avoid changing from high to low heels.
12. Put a footrail under the desk and a footrest under the crib.
13. Diaper the baby sitting next to him or her on the bed.
14. Don't stoop and stretch to hang the wash; raise the clothes basket and lower the wash line.
15. Beg or buy a rocking chair. Rocking rests the back by changing the muscle groups used.
16. Train yourself vigorously to use your abdominal muscles to flatten your lower abdomen. In time, this muscle contraction will become habitual, making you the envied possessor of a youthful body profile!

17. Don't strain to open windows or doors.
18. For good posture, concentrate on strengthening "nature's corset"—the abdominal and buttock muscles. The pelvic roll exercise is especially recommended to correct the postural relation between the pelvis and the spine.

TENDINITIS

Tendinitis or tenosynovitis is the third ailment in rowing. It refers to an inflammation of a tendon. Although tendinitis could occur anywhere on the body where there are tendons, in rowing it most frequently occurs in the forearm and occasionally in the shoulder. Quite frankly, tendinitis in the forearm rarely occurs, and when it does it usually affects people who "feather" (roll or rotate) the rowing arm.

RICE is the standard treatment for tendinitis of the forearm and shoulder. Also, to prevent tendinitis of the forearm, avoid the feathering action in rowing.

Both forearm and shoulder tendinitis start slowly. First, there is an uneasy feeling in the shoulder or forearm. Over the next 12–24 hours the pain becomes more acute. The pain is quite acute when doing the rowing motion.

As with the other injuries, tendinitis is caused by overuse—doing too much too soon, using a lever resistance that is too great, or rowing too long or too fast.

Cortisone and aspirin are standard medical therapy. A better suggestion is RICE, followed by a gradual reintroduction to rowing—with moderate resistance, pace, and duration.

9

ACCESSORIES FOR TRAINING

MOST ROWING MACHINES have few, if any, accessories. Those with accessories may have a counter and/or a timer, and that's about it. The ProForm 935, however, comes with a so-called Electronic Coxswain (see photo on page 103). The AMF Benchmark also has electronic devices.

The ProForm 935 is equipped with a microprocessor that I'm sure will become a standard component of the top-of-the-line rowers from the various companies. It is a far cry from the standard counter located on most rowers (see page 103).

ProForm's microprocessor helps you monitor the level and intensity of your workout. In measuring distance and speed, the Electronic Coxswain assumes that a racing shell is in calm water and that the average stroke length is over 14 feet. All measurements are taken from switches mounted inside the machine and are triggered by magnetic fields. There are eight keys on a keyboard and an LCD display.

The U/min displays your stroke rate, or "rating" in rowing parlance. This is your number of strokes per two-minute interval.

The Start-Stop button is a stopwatch. Fortunately, you can use any other function without interrupting the stopwatch. For example, to monitor intensity of exercise, select stroke rate. At the end of the workout, or during different intervals, press the Start-Stop button to determine the duration of exercise.

The Set-Reset button is used to clear the display and reset the various function keys.

The Max Speed button indicates your maximum rowing speed. To determine the maximum rowing speed at selected intervals or at the end of the workout, this button is pushed.

The M/S button displays the total miles rowed since the battery was installed. The battery can even be replaced without disturbing the total miles rowed.

The 0 MPH button is your average rowing speed beginning at 2 miles per hour.

T-M/S button displays the miles rowed during the current workout.

Concept II Ergometer has a computerized video output monitor for incentive and fun. Called ExerVISION, it sells for $60 and hooks up to your computer and television. The ExerVISION runs on the Commodore 64 and VIC-20.

To operate, you turn on the TV, turn on the computer, load the program, and then type "RUN." The program asks your workout format (length and speed of paces). The computer does its part as you row. It runs your complete workout for you and paces you with a little videographic boat. It shows and tells you how far ahead of or behind the pacer you are. Running time is kept on the screen along with other helpful information. At the finish, the data from your workout are posted: time, distance, average pace, watt output (work unit), approximate value for oxygen intake, and calories used.

PULSE RATE COMPUTERS

As you learned in Chapter 4, all you need to do to design an exercise program for rowing is check your pulse rate. There are, of course, some people who have a hard time counting their pulse rate, and others who don't want (or like) to count pulse during exercise. Still others do not trust their ability to count their pulse rate. If you are one of the above, you may be interested in one of the pulse rate or heart rate computers, which range in price from $60 to well over $200.

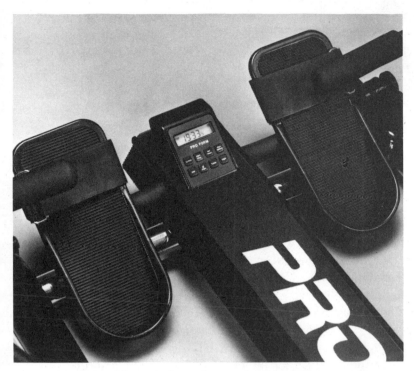

The ProForm Electronic Coxswain.

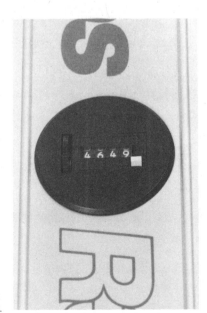

Standard stroke counter located on the
typical rowing machine.

Some of the heart rate devices attach to the finger. Some are fastened to the earlobe, and some go around your chest with a belt.

I have found that my pulse rate varies greatly when measured by the finger heart rate devices. They work well if I stay reasonably still, but when I move a great deal the readings are bizarre. My personal observations, plus reactions from many people in my fitness programs, have been substantiated by *Bicycling* magazine. The editors found that the models they tested compared favorably with the local hospital's EKG unit, provided that the user stayed reasonably still. They also found that when the person moved around or moved the fingers some meters gave readings that fluctuated as much as 60 beats. The units least affected are the ear clip or chest strap. The finger devices were found to be the least reliable.

The Genesis Exercise Computer 100 (Biometric Systems, 4040 Del Ray Ave., Marina Del Ray, CA 90291) looks like a huge electronic wristwatch. It weighs about three ounces and has a plastic housing measuring 3 by 2¼ by ⅝ inches. The face is a digital, liquid crystal readout with three touch controls and a knob for adjusting a metronome. Your pulse rate is picked up by a small band worn near the little finger or another finger. This can be a problem when gripping the rower arms and moving rapidly. The band connects to the housing on your wrist with a 7-inch wire. Two 1.5-volt batteries provide power.

The Genesis doesn't just record your pulse rate. You can set a pulse rate range, and a beeper will tell you when your rate is above or below these limits. The Genesis will also tell you how long you've kept your rate within these limits and how long it takes your pulse to settle down to a base rate that you set. There is also a built-in metronome that beeps between 60 and 120 beats per minute, depending on your wishes.

The Pulse Tach, Model S33-160 (Edmund Scientific Company, 101 E. Glouster Pike, Barrington, NJ 08007; $59.95) is a watch that has the usual features of a calendar, alarm, and chronograph stopwatch, but it also has a built-in monitor on its face. To get a readout, you put your finger on the sensor and wait until the readout stops counting.

The Pulse Tach Fingertip Heart Computer (Bay Star, 110 Painters Mill Rd., Dept. 97, Owings Mills, MD 21117) weighs about 3¾ ounces and is two inches long and one inch wide. It is a miniaturized, digital heart rate meter that fits entirely on the end of your finger. You'll need to stop rowing to use this satisfactorily. A built-in beeper lets you hear your pulse. There is a one-hour stopwatch to time your recovery and a large liquid crystal, digital display.

The Pulse Tach has an automatic shutoff, long-lasting batteries, and a lanyard to hang around your neck.

The Amerec 150 Sport Tester Telemeter uses a telemetry system that remotely transmits and receives your heart rate data while you work out.

The Sport Tester Telemeter combines an adjustable chest harness and heart rate transmitter with a receiver that can be handheld, attached to the wrist, or slipped into the harness holder. This is a short-range telemetry only, about three feet.

The Sport Tester, in addition to monitoring heart rate, can be used as a multifunction programmable training aid. It helps you make the most of your workout by letting you set upper and lower limit alarms at the desired heart rates to keep you working within your training zone. The Amerec 150 also functions as a stopwatch and a clock with a programmable alarm feature. The field transmitter weighs only 1½ ounces, and the microcomputer receiver weighs only 1 ounce.

The TE 2000 Sport Tester (made in Finland, distributed by AMF American Inc., 200 American Ave., Jefferson, IA 50129; $250) is like the Amerec 150. It uses radio technology to beam your pulse into a small wristwatch monitor. The monitor picks up the signal from a rubber chest strap that contains electrodes similar to those used with ECG machines. There are no wires.

The Sport Tester provides information on regular time, elapsed time, and average pulse as well as moment-to-moment readout on where the heart is headed.

The 1-2-3 Heart Rate Monitor (Country Technology Inc., PO Box 85, Gays Mills, WI 54631; $295) is a new heart rate meter that delivers supposedly quick, accurate readings without a confusing display of false readings. The first reading (after three rhythmic heart signals) is supposedly accurate. The heart rate monitor uses a new ECG electro-sensor that seems to handle perspiration, body oils, and motion. To use the device, you do not need to wear a chest strap harness. You simply place one finger of each hand on the sensors. A four-beat average heart rate is quickly displayed. There is an automatic turnoff and a liquid crystal display.

The Activmeter (Country Technology, Inc., PO Box 87, Gays Mills, WI 54631; $90) is worn on the wrist like a watch and senses the pulse rate with a photo-optic finger sensor. Upper and lower limits activate a warning tone to keep the level of exercise in the proper training range. Heart rate measures are updated every seven to eight seconds. A time function is also incorporated to time either exercise duration or cardiac recovery time.

The Exersentry Heart Rate Monitor (Respironics, Inc., 650 Seco Rd., Monroeville, PA 15146; $185, $17.50 for bike mounting, $15 for 36-inch cable) uses conductive rubber-sensing electrodes that require no gels. The electrodes fasten to a chest belt and rely on the skin's moisture to sense the heart's electrical system. The Exersentry has a beeper with upper and lower alarm limits, so you can exercise within your training zone. The Exersentry remains quiet as long as the heart rate remains within the training zone. A miniature earphone is also available to block out surrounding noise interference. The heart rate display ranges from 40 to over 200 beats per minute. The weight of the device is three ounces. The electrode belt weighs 6½ ounces. The device measures 4 by 2.5 by 1 inch. It requires one 1.5-volt, AAA alkaline battery.

The Amerec 160 Vital Signs Monitor (Amerec, PO Box 3825, Bellevue, WA 98009; $295) provides a printed record of systolic and diastolic blood pressures, heart rate, and body temperature along with the date and time of the readings.

The Amerec 160 has a built-in programmable reminder signal that can be set to alert you to take your measurements at a particular time of the day.

Blood pressure and pulse are taken using the traditional inflation cuff and squeeze bulb, only the function is automatic. Body temperature is measured by a thermal probe, under either the tongue or the armpit.

The compact and lightweight monitor can be powered by batteries for maximum flexibility.

The Coach Model S33-106 (Biotechnology, Inc., 6924 NW 46th St., Miami, FL 33166; $199.95) uses a chest strap with electrodes, with a wire that runs from the strap to a minicomputer. The minicomputer clips on to your waistband. The readout runs along the top of the monitor. When you wear it while running you can measure your distance, calories burned, number of strides, average speed, and elapsed time. While you are wearing the chest strap it measures your heart rate and will beep when you exceed your preset target pulse rate. You can program it to your needs by punching in data on your sex, age, weight, and resting and target maximum heart rates.

THE CHRONOGRAPH: THE EXERCISERS' WATCH

Chronographs are the watches of the '80s. They are big business. Most people into exercise are avid chronograph users. Chronographs are perfect for anyone who is exercising. You can use it to determine your performance based on time. The chronograph is a stopwatch to carry on your wrist, but it also contains many other features such as pacing, time, and alarm.

In their January 1984 issue, the editors of *Runner's World* evaluated the chronographs. The chart is reproduced on page 108, with the addresses for obtaining the products on page 109.

More than a dozen companies market chronographs. But virtually all the circuits come from Switzerland and Japan. According to the *Runner's World* group, the Accusplit 934 Turbo is the most sophisticated on the market. It seems to do everything but stand on its own head. Not only does it give you the traditional things such as alarm, light for night use, day and time, etc., but it can also provide a count-down and count-up time, calculate the elapsed time for a particular distance without erasing the running time. Even if you know the total distance you are going to go and the split distance, you can project your finish time.

Table 16:
Chronographs*

	Compo-sition	Ease of switch-ing modes	Weight	Reada-bility	Sturdi-ness	Com-fort	Over-all Rating	Price	Photo No.
Accusplit 930XP	P	8.3	8	9.3	8.3	9	8.5	$39.95	71 (70*)
Accusplit 943Turbo	P	8.5	7.5	9.5	8.5	8	8.4	$89.95	72 (71*)
Accusplit 932XP	P	8.5	7.5	9.5	8.5	8	8.4	$49.95	73 (72*)
RDA Runmaster	P	8.4	7.4	9.5	7.3	7.2	5.9	$79.95	
Accusplit 920L	P	6	8.5	6.5	8	9	7.6	$29.95	
Seiko Training Timer	M	8.2	6.6	7.2	8.4	7.4	7.56	$95.00	
Casio J-50	P	5.8	8.5	8	7.5	7.8	7.52	$29.95	
Cronus W-Watch	P	8	9	6	7	7.5	7.4	$39.95	
Innovative Pulse Watch	P	8	7.3	7	6.8	6.5	7.1	$74.95	
Casio J-30	P	7.6	7.6	6.8	6.4	6.6	7	$24.95	
Innovative Ladies' Champion	P	5.5	8.6	5.8	6.6	8.2	6.94	$29.95	74 (73*)
Innovative Men's Mariner	P	6.6	7	7.7	6.3	7	6.92	$29.95	75 (74*)
Pulsar KB003S	P	8	7.3	6.8	6	6	6.84	$49.50	
Accusplit 920XP	P	7	8	6	7	6	6.8	$29.95	76 (75*)
Timex 67731	P	4.5	8.6	5.6	6.8	8.2	6.74	$27.95	
Chronosport Navigator	P	7.8	4.3	8.8	8	4.8	6.74	$135.00	

Key:　P　= Plastic　　　Scale 1–10:　1 = unacceptable
　　　M = Metal　　　　　　　　　　10 = acceptable

Accusplit, 2290A Ringwood Ave., San Jose, CA 95131; (800) 538-9750

Biotechnology Inc., 6924 NW 46th St., Miami, FL 33166; (305) 592-6069

Bay Star Merchandise, 110 Painters Mill Rd., Owings Mills, MD 21117; (301) 363-4304

Casio, Inc., 15 Gardner Rd., Fairfield, NJ 07006; (201) 575-7400

Chronosport, Inc., 47 Walker St., Norwalk, CT 06854; (203) 853-9593

Computer Instruments Corp., 100 Madison Ave., Hempstead, NY 11550; (516) 483-8200

Cronus Precision Products, 2895 Northwestern Pkwy., Santa Clara, CA 95051; (408) 988-2500

Digital Devices, Inc., 3 Ash Place, Huntington, NY 11743; (516) 549-8585

Innovative Time Corp., 6054 Corte del Cedro, Carlsbad, CA 92008; (619) 438-0595

Medana Watch Corp., 44 E. 32nd St., New York, NY 10016; (212) 889-3560

Omega Watch Corp., 301 E. 57th St., New York, NY 10022; (212) 753-3000

On the Run, 107 Roberts St., Fargo, ND 58102; (701) 232-9400

Pulsar Time Inc., 111 MacArthur Blvd., Mahwah, NJ 07430; (201) 335-5199

Seiko, 640 5th Ave., New York, NY 10019; (212) 977-2800

Timex, Box 2126, Waterbury, CT 06720; (203) 573-5000

10

WHERE TO BUY ROWING MACHINES

SEVERAL COMPANIES SUPPLY rowing machines. The following names and addresses make up only a partial list. These companies provide rowing machines and associated components.

AJAY
1501 E. Wisconsin St.
Delavan, WI 53115

Allegheny International
  Exercise Company
US 321 Bypass North
Lincolnton, NC 28093

Amerec Corp.
PO Box 3825
Bellevue, WA 98009

AMF-American
200 American Ave.
Jefferson, IA 50129

Atlantic Fitness Products
170-A Penrod Ct.
Glen Burnie, MD 21061

Battle Creek Equipment
307 W. Jackson St.
Battle Creek, MI 49016

Concept II
RFD 2, Box 6410
Morrisville, VT 05661

The Sharper Image
680 Davis St.
San Francisco, CA 94111

Diversified Products
309 Williamson Ave.
Opelika, AL 36802

PROFORM
8170 SW Nimbus
Beaverton, OR 97005-6423

Fitness Products
PO Box 254
Hillsdale, MI 49242

Roadmaster Corp.
AMF-Wheel Good
Olney, IL 62450

M & R Industries, Inc.
9215 151st Ave., NE
Redmond, WA 98052

Vitamaster Industries
455 Smith St.
Brooklyn, NY 11231

MacLevy Product Corp.
43–23 91st Pl.
Elmhurst, NY 11373

Walton Manufacturing Co.
106 Regal Rd.
Dallas, TX 75247

PreCor
9449 151st Ave., NE
Redmond, WA 98052

Rowing machines may also be purchased from chain stores such as Montgomery Ward; Sears, Roebuck and Co.; J. C. Penney; K-Mart; Herman's; and from local sporting goods stores and discount houses.

APPENDIX

Home Gym Workout
Rowing Record

Day/ Time	Resting Pulse Rate	Rating Strokes/ min.	mph/kph (Optional)	Resist- ance	Minutes Exercised	Exercise Pulse Rate	Comments

Appendix (cont.):
Home Gym Workout
Rowing Record

Day/ Time	Resting Pulse Rate	Rating Strokes/ min.	mph/kph (Optional)	Resist- ance	Minutes Exercised	Exercise Pulse Rate	Comments